"The plutocrats who profit from the medical industry don't want you to know that there is a simple mixture of common North American herbs that shows great potential for the treatment of cancer, a disease which provides the medical establishment with megadoses of money."

—*The Spotlight*

"In this compact and intelligently presented book, Cynthia Olsen goes a long way toward giving Essiac its proper due "as perhaps not a universal cure but a recognized remedy" in the treatment of cancer. [This book] provides the historical context of this herbal treatment along with a materia medica on the four herbs that make up Essiac. Olsen never bullies her readers. Instead, she provides enough information so that the individual can make his or her own decisions regarding use of Essiac. In this vein, Olsen correctly, I think, provides a framework for working with herbs (as opposed to pharmaceutical drugs) in the treatment of disease."

—*Small Press*

"The author does a good job of reviewing the history of this formula as well as scientific reasons why these herbs may affect the growth of cancer cells or support the immune system. Unlike others who have written books about Essiac, Olsen takes the time to discuss what is known about the Ojibwa healers and how their traditional methods may have resulted in this tea."

—*Common Ground*

"*Essiac: A Native Herbal Cancer Remedy*, winner of the 1997 Small Press Book Award, is an insightful account of the history and applications of this time-proven natural Canadian herbal remedy. Author Cynthia B. Olsen offers insight into the restorative properties of Essiac and the necessity of harmony between spirit, mind and body that can be obtained through exercise, meditation and herbal medication. This complete work offers information about nutrition and exercise that is vital to everyone, even those not experiencing ailments."

—*The Edge*

Winner of
Small Press Book Award
in
Health, Medicine and Nutrition

ESSIAC

A Native Herbal Cancer Remedy

— 2nd Edition —

Cynthia Olsen

with contributions by
Dr. Jim Chan & Christopher Gussa

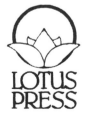

LOTUS
PRESS

Twin Lakes, Wisconsin

DISCLAIMER:
Some of the manufacturers are stating that their formula is the best and the most authentic. Please take with "a grain of salt" what people may tell you about the merits of their products. It is vitally important for each person who may be ill with cancer or any disease to seek their own counsel by going within before deciding on course of action. In spite of all the positive testimony, Essiac should not be considered a universal cure for cancer. The results vary from case to case. The herbs burdock, sheep sorrel, turkey rhubarb, and slippery elm have excellent properties that will assist the body in strengthening the immune system as well as in cleansing and assisting various organs to function properly.

First published in 1996, revised in 1998 by Kali Press
Second US Edition published by:
Lotus Press, PO Box 325, Twin Lakes, WI 53181
Email: lotuspress@lotuspress.com
Website: www.lotuspress.com

Library of Congress Cataloging-in-Publication Data
Olsen, Cynthia
        Essiac: a native herbal cancer remedy / Cynthia Olsen, with
    contributions by Jim Chan & Christopher Gussa. — 2nd ed.
            p.   cm.
    Includes bibliographical references and index.
    ISBN: 978-1-8909-4100-0
        1. Essiac—Therapeutic use. 2. Cancer—Alternative treatment.
    3. Burdocks—Therapeutic use. 4. Sheep sorrel—Therapeutic use.
    5. Turkey rhubarb—Therapeutic use. 6. Slippery elm—Therapeutic
    use. I. Chan, Jim. II. Gussa, Christopher. III. Title
    RC271.
E68047   1998   98-35978
    616.99 ' 406—DC21
CIP

Editing, contribution and illustrations of Essiac herbs: Peter Marritt
Design and additional illustrations: Paul Bond, Art & Soul Design
Cover photograph of Burdock Root: Stephen Foster
Five Rites photographs: Preston Sowell
Five Rites model: Courtney M. Hill
Cover photograph of Midiwiwin Medicine Man by permission from the Smithsonian Enthological Archives
Photograph of Rene Caisse by permission from the Bracebridge Library, Bracebridge, Ontario, Canada -photo property of Mary Macpherson

Printed in the United States of America

TRIBUTE TO JENI ERICSON KYLEIGH

April 8, 1932 - May 31, 1998

*To my special friend Jeni Ericson Kyleigh
who made her transition on May 31, 1998.
You will be greatly missed.
Your spirit essence will always remain in our hearts.*

ACKNOWLEDGEMENTS

*I have deep gratitude for all the people who
contributed their time, efforts and creative
processes to help make this book possible.*

*To my dear friend, Jeni, who planted the seed to make
this project come to life;*

*To Peter Marritt, not only for editing the work,
but contributing his worthwhile ideas to make
the book more complete in form;*

*Paul Bond, for making the book come alive with
his artistic cover design and layout;*

*To my lovely daughter, Courtney, for taking the time
to pose for the five rites, and Preston Sowell
for doing such a fine job photographing her;*

*Rick Sibley, for countless hours
of research and compiling data;*

*Sue Tinkle, for editing contribution,
and Paige Mooy for herb research;*

*To Rene Caisse and the Ojibwa Indians for
their knowledge, humility and dedication in
their work with these herbs.*

*Most of all, to Spirit who has guided and shown me my
willingness to be of service once again.*

CONTENTS

CAUTION AND DISCLAIMER

Unquestionably, many have been helped by Essiac. Rene Caisse, the Canadian nurse who perfected the formula, successfully treated thousands during more than 50 years of a practice that engendered considerable controversy. Almost 400 people were ready to testify at a Cancer Commission hearing in Toronto in 1939 that they had been restored to health by Essiac. Often those who were helped by this simple herbal tea tried it as a last resort after little or no success with conventional methods. And, unlike mainstream therapies, the mixture seems totally harmless and non-toxic. Each of the herbs in Essiac has been used as food.

It must be emphasized, however, that Essiac may not help you, your friend, or your loved one with cancer. We live in complicated, challenging times amid an increasingly toxic environment. We are also learning that stress, along with mental and emotional imbalance, may be the real cause of much dis-ease.

Our task was simply to compile and present some of the available information about the basic herbal formula called Essiac. The name Essiac, is simply Caisse spelled backwards.

The information contained in this book is a compilation of research, data, testimonials and related subject matter on Essiac. The information provided here is a general guide for the individual. Each person should consult with his or her doctor for treatment.

In 1900 the death rate from cancer was 63 per 100,000 people. In 1926, the rate rose to 103 per 100,000 people. In 1993, cancer claimed the lives of over half a million people in the U.S. alone. The American Cancer Society has stated that in 1996 a million and a half people were diagnosed with some kind of cancer; prostate cancer being the number one cancer among men, while breast cancer is the highest among women. Although there are a multitude of factors that may create cancer, there isn't a magic bullet that can deal with cancer.

Essiac is to be viewed as not a universal cure but a recognized historic use of herbs.

FOREWORD

*H*omo sapiens, also known as human, is a very peculiar species. Indeed, if there were another species capable of achieving the same level of intelligence and civilization, the study of the human could be their hottest topic. While most living beings are either designed or prepared to face their destiny, humans live in denial of death. In the near perfect society of bees, drones are killed after their jobs are done; workers are sterilized so that they can concentrate on their jobs. When faced with the shortage of food, the high level of stress triggers rats to commit mass suicide by jumping off a cliff.

The day a human is born, he/she is destined to face death. In our present society, one of the most common causes of death is cancer. Cancer is a consequence of the failure of the repairing and defense mechanisms of our body. In a sense it is the ultimate failure of the functional aspects of an organism. Yet we pour billions of dollars (a representation of massive effort) into trying to overcome this failure. Can our destiny be avoided? At best we may buy a postponement.

All the destructive interventions against cancer have brought us nothing more than disappointments. Many apparently safe and effective remedies have either been laughed at or neglected since the formation of the American Medical Association, even though the present conventional medical profession is struggling to come to terms with the validity of what they used to make a mockery of. The process may be just a few steps too slow for some of us who are striving to defy cancer's natural progression so we can be with our loved ones for one more day.

Much of our effort is spent in validating the most obvious, such as the vitamin C project of the National Institute of Health (NIH); remedies such as the Hoxsey formula, the Burton immune augmentation therapy, the Livingston Wheeler immunotherapy, the Revicci therapy, the Pridden BCT therapy, Dr. Bryzinsky's Anti-neoplastin, Dr. Kelly's enzyme therapy, and the list goes on. One of these is Rene Caisse's Essiac. Ms. Caisse spent a good part of her life working on Essiac. Dr. Ralph Moss, PhD, who was a scientific writer for the Memorial Sloan Kettering Center, can tell you in his writings about how Ms. Caisse was treated by the authorities. Ms. Caisse had indeed brought to mankind a unique opportunity, a second chance to learn the lessons of life and death.

In this book, Cynthia Olsen will walk us through the history and development of Essiac (the word Caisse spelled backwards). We might well look at Essiac as symbolizing the reversal of the degenerative process.

Dr. Jim Chan (Bastyr)
at Vancouver, B.C., Canada
January 1996

Introduction

"I endorse this therapy even today

for I have in fact cured my own cancer,

the original site of which was the lower bowel,

through ESSIAC alone."

Dr. Charles Brusch, M.D.,
President John F. Kennedy's personal physician

$\mathcal{I}$ first met Jeni at a yard sale that was being held at a nearby campground. She had arrived in our peaceful mountain town the week before... Jeni had fled Sedona, Arizona after a major rainstorm had created the waters of Oak Creek to rise and flood many homes close by. Jeni was house sitting at a home that was situated very near the creek. She managed to grab some of her belongings, but in the process, had lost many of her art pieces and weavings that were part of her livelihood.

It was July 4th when we first met. I was on my way to a picnic, when I spotted a 'campground sale' sign which caught my eye. I swung into the parking area. Walking down the line of tables, I stepped in front of one which had spiritual music, linens, candles and some clothes. I recall her standing there. She was rather tall and slim with shortly cropped blonde hair. Her smile was contagious and her talk animated. For some-time we conversed, and then she invited me to sit in one of the folding chairs next to her. She proceeded to tell me how she arrived in town and came across the campground where she was temporarily staying until she could find more permanent housing. One thing led to another, and I invited Jeni to come live with me for awhile until she found her own place.

During the next five years of our mutually fulfilling friendship, Jeni and I talked about her challenges fighting her breast cancer. She had been diagnosed with the illness for about 3 years at that time. She elected not to seek mainstream (allopathic) medical care or expose her body to destructive treatments such as surgery, chemotherapy or radiation. Instead she was convinced she could cure herself using natural ways which included herbs, juices, eliminating red meat, receiving bodywork and other complementary modalities. Her mother also had breast cancer and decided to be treated with the traditional method of chemotherapy and radiation. Jeni had witnessed the pain her mother had gone through and so when she was diagnosed with breast cancer as well, she decided not to choose the same path her mother had taken. Jeni had also shared with me that perhaps the most important part of her therapy involved her emotional well being. She recognized the impact of early childhood feelings of rejection and felt that her complete healing may well depend upon accepting all her feelings and loving herself for the perfect being that she is and always has been.

I began to get a feeling of what it must have been like for Rene Caisse to devotedly brew up thousands of mixtures over a fifty year period while observing Jeni in my kitchen cooking the herbs in large pots. The room would fill with the steam and smells of a mixture that may have originated with the Ojibwa (Chippewa) Indians of the Lake Country in Canada. I tried it myself and found the taste quite soothing, especially before retiring in the evening. Jeni took the tea twice daily, and it really seemed to keep her stamina high and ward off illnesses.

As I became more and more intrigued with Jeni's quest, I decided to research the information on this formula. I discovered that although the clinical data was sketchy to say the least, the volume of positive testimony is impressive. The many articles and stories about Essiac also attest to Rene Caisse's devotion and effort, as well as her success. She administered the treatment completely free of charge to thousands of patients.

I learned that there is considerable mystery surrounding the Essiac formula. A full blooded Ojibwa (Sault St. Marie Chippewa) who is a professor of Native American Studies at a western university, informed me that the tribal medicine society, which calls itself the Midewiwin, is extremely secretive. Perhaps there are other herbs that are used for different types of cancer. Maybe the formula Rene Caisse learned of was a specific remedy for a particular patient. The Midewiwin no doubt use herbs that are indigenous to their region and call upon their spirit guides and intuition as well as their training and experience to assist them in deciding which particular plants would benefit each person being treated.

Caisse herself was secretive about the formula. She knew it worked and was apparently concerned that it be made available immediately and inexpensively to any who needed it. As you will learn in Chapter 1, she struggled for years against a medical establishment intensely jealous of its lucrative turf as well as a governmental bureaucracy intent on their red-tape-riddled procedures. It seems that her only desire was that the people who need help would get it.

It's been reported that Nurse Caisse experienced a recovery rate of over 80%. How much of this was due to the positive and nurturing atmosphere at her clinic is anybody's guess. Those were simpler times. In this day and age, stress, skepticism, and our increasingly toxic environment all conspire against our quest for the complete cure. In the last year of her life, Rene finally sold the formula to the Resperin Corporation of Ontario, Canada, for $1.00.

You will find instructions for the preparation of the Essiac formula in Chapter 5. Although this is the most economical approach, it is time consuming.

I met Christopher Gussa who is the founder of the Desert Dragon Healing Center in Tucson, Arizona. He is a Clinical Herbalist and Chinese Practitioner. Chris has used fresh whole herbs and combined them with his own pills, extracts, syrups and other formulas. In chapter eight, Gussa discusses his experience with the Ojibwa herbs and the use of Blood Root. I believe the readers will find this chapter enlightening and inspiring.

There are also several manufacturers of products that contain the herbs premixed and ready to take. Some of these products are sold in health food stores throughout North America in capsule form, liquid, a tincture, and soon, a powder. A few of these are detailed in the Resources section at the end of the book.

It's important to recognize the body, mind, spirit connection in addressing the illness. Diet, exercise, visualization, stress reduction, meditation and getting in touch with the vital energy force of one's being should all be given consideration. Please read the information in this book with a discerning eye. Educate yourself so that you can discover the direction which most closely 'resonates' with you for your particular condition. In other words, follow your own heart - your own intuition.

Cynthia Olsen
Pagosa Springs, Colorado
June 1998

CHAPTER ONE

The History of Essiac

"A holy drink that would purify

her body and place it back in balance

with the Great Spirit."

Rene Caisse's description of the Ojibwa medicine man's
original description of Essiac to the English woman who
gave Caisse the formula in 1922.

*I*n 1922, Rene Caisse made a discovery that changed her life dramatically. While attending to an older woman who had had surgery, Nurse Caisse noticed scarring on the woman's breast and asked her how it came about. The woman explained that 30 years earlier she had developed breast cancer and had been led to an old Indian medicine man who told her the cancer could be cured with an herbal remedy that he knew of. After a disappointing visit to a doctor, she decided to go back to the Indian who gave her an herbal formula and instructions on how to brew it. She drank the herbal mixture daily, and within time the breast tumors gradually diminished. She never had a recurrence and was 80 years old at the time Rene Caisse met her.

Caisse asked the woman for the formula, saying that: "My thought was that if I should ever develop cancer, I would use it." About a year after this incident, she "was visiting a retired doctor, whom I knew well. We were walking slowly about his garden when he took his cane and lifted a weed. `Nurse Caisse,' he told me, `if people would use this weed there would be little or no cancer in the world.' It was one of the plants my patient had named as an ingredient of the Indian medicine man's tea!"

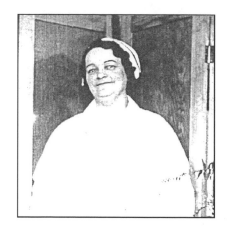

Rene Caisse
1888 - 1978

She did little with the Essiac formula until 1924 when her aunt developed stomach and liver cancer. The doctors had given her aunt six months to live. Rene obtained permission from her aunt's physician, Dr. R. O. Fisher, to administer the herbal tea treatment. Rene later said, "My aunt lived for twenty-one years after being given up by the medical profession. There was no recurrence of cancer."

> "My aunt lived for twenty-one years after being given up by the medical profession. There was no recurrence of cancer."

Caisse and Dr. Fisher began experimenting with the Essiac treatment in a makeshift lab in her mother's basement. In 1925 Dr. Fisher suggested Essiac inoculation for quicker results in addition to giving the treatment orally. The first human inoculation was given to a man with cancer of the throat and tongue. In Rene's words: "I was nearly scared to death. There was a violent reaction. The patient developed a severe chill; his tongue swelled so badly the doctor had to press it down with a spatula to let him breathe. This lasted about twenty minutes. Then the swelling went down, the chill subsided, and the patient was all right. The cancer stopped growing, the patient went home, and lived quite comfortably for almost four years."

In 1926, a group of eight doctors asked Rene to treat an old man who had cancer and was expected to live only ten days. After the treatment, the man lived six months. The same eight doctors signed and sent a petition to the capitol in Ottawa asking the government to provide Caisse with treatment facilities. The petition was denied, and Caisse was threatened with arrest. She was not arrested because she did not charge fees and she worked under the auspices of the doctors.

Between 1928 and 1930, Dr. W. C. Arnold, one of the doctors sent by the governmental investigation, was so impressed with her results that he asked Caisse to perform research on mice with Essiac, as the herbal tea treatment was now commonly called. She was given space at the Christie Street Hospital Laboratories under the supervision of Drs. Norich and Lockhead. The mice were injected with Rous Sarcoma, and then treated with Essiac. The mice lived for fifty-two days, longer than with any other treatment.

In 1929, Rene Caisse, feeling a persecution that would haunt her throughout her career, gave up professional nursing which was consuming twelve hours a day. She devoted her time to Essiac research, and in her apartment in Bracebridge, Ontario began treating thirty patients each day. That year she met Dr. Frederick Banting of the Banting Institute, Department of Medical Research, University of Toronto. Dr. Banting is the co- discoverer of insulin for diabetes. Dr Banting knew of a woman who was diabetic and had cancer of the colon. During her Essiac treatments she didn't take any insulin. After her recovery, she had no signs of diabetes. Dr. Banting stated that "Essiac had somehow stimulated the pancreas to function normally, thereby healing the diabetes."

Dr. Banting reviewed Rene's case studies including pictures before and after treatments, and said, "Miss Caisse, I will not say you have a cure for cancer, but you have more evidence of a beneficial treatment for cancer than anyone in the world." Banting invited her to continue her research at the University of Toronto; however, she would have to disclose the formula for Essiac, and she was apparently concerned that the remedy would either be suppressed or not used properly and economically. She declined the offer and went back to Bracebridge, Ontario to continue treating patients.

> "Miss Caisse, I will not say you have a cure for cancer, but you have more evidence of a beneficial treatment for cancer than anyone in the world."

In 1930 the Canadian College of Physicians and Surgeons sent an agent to issue a warrant for Rene Caisse's arrest for practicing medicine without a license. When the agent discovered Caisse was not only providing free services but also working only with permission and approval from doctors, the warrant was never served.

CAISSE'S WORK ACKNOWLEDGED

A 1932 headline in the *Toronto Star* read, "Bracebridge Girl Makes Notable Discovery Against Cancer." Ironically, this story brought on another threat of arrest and imprisonment for practicing medicine without a license. At age forty-four, already mentally and physically over-stressed, Rene was granted a hearing with the Canadian Minister of Health, The Honorable Dr. J. A. Faulkner. She was accompanied by patients and supporting doctors, and after hearing the evidence, Dr. Faulkner allowed her to continue with Essiac treatments providing she did not charge a fee and had a doctor's written diagnosis.

Because of the notoriety Caisse received for her wonderful work, the Bracebridge Town Council donated the old, deserted British Lion Hotel building to be used for patient treatment. She now had five treatment rooms, an office, a dispensary and a reception area. For eight years, until 1942, thousands of people came for treatments; most were severely ill with cancer.

Rene Caisse's mother was diagnosed with liver cancer in 1935. An internationally known doctor, Roscoe Graham, informed her that her mother had just "days to live." Rene never told her mother of the cancer, but treated her with Essiac for ten days, slowly reducing the dosage. Her mother recovered completely and lived another eighteen years until her death at age ninety of heart failure.

Two more petitions signed by prominent physicians on Caisse's behalf were presented in 1936 to Canadian authorities urging facilities be provided and credence given to Essiac. There was no response to either petition.

In that same year the Alumni Association of Northwestern University near Chicago notified Dr. John Wolfer of the medical school of Caisse's treatment efforts and persuaded him to meet with her to discuss terminally ill patients. Rene agreed to treat patients each week under the observation of five doctors.

The treatments went well, and she was offered a clinic Passervant Hospital in Chicago. She was also offered an opportunity to work with Dr. Richard Leonardo, a specialist from Rochester, New York. Leonardo was skeptical at first: "You're doing them [patients] good, but it's your personality and the hope you offer them [that gets the results]." Later, after reviewing treatment results and talking with patients, Leonardo said, "Well, by God, you've got it! But the medical profession isn't going to let you do this to me. I've spent seven years in medical school, and I've written books."

Caisse declined both offers, not only because she would have had to divulge Essiac's formula and thus run the risk that it would not be used, but also because she felt an obligation and responsibility to her patients and the Canadian people.

The next year, in 1937, Dr. Emma M. Carson, a Los Angeles physician, visited Bracebridge and wrote a favorable report on Caisse and her clinic. "I was firmly resolved that my investigation be based on unprejudiced judgment. The vast majority of Miss Caisse's patients were brought to her after surgery, radiation, x-rays, emplastrums, etc. had failed to be helpful and the patients were pronounced incurable or hopeless cases. The progress obtainable and the actual results from Essiac treatments, and the rapidity of repair were absolutely marvelous, and must have been seen to be believed. My skepticism neither yielded nor became subdued by the hopes and faith so definitely expressed by the patients and their friends. As I reviewed, compared and summarized my data, records, case histories, etc., I realized that skepticism had deserted me. When I arrived, I contemplated remaining 12 hours - I remained 24 days. I examined results obtained on 400 patients."

> **"The progress obtainable and the actual results from Essiac treatments, and the rapidity of repair were absolutely marvelous, and must have been seen to be believed."**

In 1938 Rene Caisse's supporters attempted to get a bill passed to give her the right to treat cancer patients without the constant threat of arrest. The bill in part would read: ". . . an act to authorize Rene Caisse to practice medicine in the Province of Ontario in the treatment of cancer and conditions resulting therefrom." The bill was initiated in the Ontario Parliament supported by a petition with over 55,000 signatures. The bill failed by three votes, and it seemed obvious at the time that it failed principally because of collusion by the Canadian Medical Association and the newly formed Cancer Commission.

Public Hearings
and Condemnation

In March 1939, a public hearing was held by the Cancer Commission at the Royal York Hotel in Toronto. Caisse brought 387 patients to testify. The Commission only heard 49 patients that Rene had treated. Patients testified to the burns from radium and the diagnosis from their doctors giving them a short time to live, all before they saw Rene Caisse. The Commission stated: "It is the opinion that the evidence adduced does not justify any favorable conclusion as to the merit of Essiac as a remedy for cancer." Rene Caisse refused to give the Commission the formula for Essiac unless they would admit the treatments she gave with Essiac had merit.

In 1942, Rene Caisse suffered a nervous collapse and decided to close her Bracebridge Clinic and move to her husband's home town of North Bay. She virtually dropped out of public view. Her husband died in 1943 of pneumonia. Little is known of Caisse's activities between her husband's death and 1958. Presumedly she treated a few seriously ill cancer patients, but the extent of that involvement is unknown.

In 1958 the Cancer Commission recommended that College of Physicians and Surgeons look into Caisse's activities. As the result of letters from patients and supporters, the Canadian premier requested that Caisse provide the commission with the formula for Essiac. She refused, citing again that if the medical world would acknowledge and administer Essiac, she would divulge the formula.

The Secretary of the Commission for the Investigation of Cancer Remedies, C. J. Telfer, wrote to the Minister of Health, Dr. Mackinnon Phillips: "At a meeting of the Commission, a letter was read from Miss Caisse, the nurse from Bracebridge who refused many years ago to divulge the formula which she was then and apparently still using in the treatment of cancer. The Commission feels no action should be taken by them, but directed the matter be brought to your attention in case you might want to refer this one also to the College [of Physicians and Surgeons]."

Premier Leslie Frost received supportive letters from Rene Caisse's patients, and Frost wrote to Rene: "It would speed matters up greatly if you would get in touch with Dr. W. G. Brown, Deputy Minister of Health, and arrange through him to give the Cancer Remedies Investigation Commission the details of your methods, so the Commission could give them a thorough analysis."

In October of 1958, Rene Caisse wrote a letter to Dr. Brown stating that it had been requested by Leslie Frost that she contact him about her Essiac treatments. Dr. McPhedran of the College of Physicians and Surgeons had ordered her to stop giving treatments. Caisse went on to say that her treatments had continued successfully because she simply could not turn away people. Several months later the College de-

> "Caisse went on to say that her treatments had continued successfully because she simply could not turn people away."

cide not to prosecute Rene Caisse and that her activities be kept under surveillance.

Ralph Daigh, an Editor with Fawcett Publishing, brought attention back to Caisse in 1959 when he arranged to have Essiac investigated by a major Boston hospital. He believed he had concrete evidence that the medical establishment had suppressed information about the efficacy of Essiac. Through Daigh's efforts, Caisse worked with Dr. Charles Brusch, John F. Kennedy's personal physician. Brusch, in turn, had the clout to interest the Sloan-Kettering Cancer Institute. Caisse's relationship with Sloan-Kettering offered the first genuine opportunity to get Essiac to the world. Unfortunately, a familiar stumbling block emerged. Fearing Essiac would be shelved if she released the formula, Caisse refused to make any deals and went back to Canada. It was speculated at the time that the AMA had a hand in Sloan-Kettering's reluctance to sponsor the treatment.

> **"He beleived he had concrete evidence that the medical establishment had suppressed information about the efficiacy of Essiac."**

Years later, in 1989, Dr. Brusch made the statement: "I still take it myself. I successfully treated my own cancer with it." He regretted that John F. Kennedy did not live long enough to help influence the medical establishment in using Essiac throughout the medical organization. One of the Brusch Clinic's "cures" involved a man who had basal cell carcinoma of the right cheek. After four treatments orally and through injections, the lesion gradually healed. The Brusch clinic called this case a "cure."

Dr. Brusch convinced the Sloan-Kettering Cancer Institute to conduct tests on animals using Essiac. They cited "...a tendency of the cancer cells to amalgamate and localize." The institute refused to continue testing unless the formula was revealed to them. Testing came to a halt. Dr. Brusch may have been the first physician with enough national notoriety who had a significant chance to get Essiac to the cancer patients who needed it on a global basis. There can be no doubt he personally believed in Essiac. He stated, "The results we obtained with thousands of patients of various races, sexes and ages with all types of cancer definitely prove Essiac to be a cure for cancer. Studies done in four laboratories in the United States and one or more in Canada also fortify this claim."

> **"The results we obtained with thousands of patients of various races, sexes and ages with all types of cancer definitely prove Essiac to be a cure for cancer."**

Later in life, Brusch developed cancer and cured it with Essiac. He stated in 1990 that, "I have taken Essiac every day since my diagnosis [1984] and my recent examination has given me a clear bill of health."

Caisse Seeks Mainstream Support

Throughout the 1960's and 1970's Rene Caisse approached several pharmaceutical companies to convince them to become involved with Essiac. The only stipulation, naturally, was that Essiac be put to immediate use with cancer patients. However, without an actual formula and without being able to conduct their own tests, none of the companies were interested.

In 1973, Rene Caisse Sloan-Kettering one last chance. Dr. Chester Stock asked Rene to send over some herbs for testing. She sent the burdock root, which seemed to have the properties of a tumor regressor. She also provided instructions on how to inject the herb. In 1975, Dr. Stock wrote to Rene and suggested that there was "regression of sarcoma 180 in mice treated with Essiac." Rene was later told, however, that test results were negative.

> **"She learned that Sloan-Kettering had not followed her instructions carefully and had frozen the herb."**

She learned that Sloan-Kettering had not followed her instructions carefully and had frozen the herb. Dr. Stock testified at a hearing that the Essiac did not perform satisfactorily on the mice and that "....we were never provided full information about the nature of Essiac." In disgust, Caisse broke all ties with Sloan-Kettering.

In 1977, shortly before Rene's death, she decided to sell her formula to the Resperin Corporation in Toronto. She also gave the Essiac formula to two friends: Mary Macpherson and Gilbert Blondin. Blondin faced a trial in 1990 for a product he developed called "Easy-Ac" with Dr. Pierre Gaulin, an American doctor. Resperin confronted them and said they were selling the Essiac illegally. Gaulin was quoted as saying "Essiac has never been shown to harm anyone in any way. I don't cure anybody. I don't perform miracles, but whatever period of life a person has to live, we should make it as easy for them as we can." It is principally through these two that the public knows the formula. Caisse also signed over the formula to Dr. Brusch almost as a dying wish.

Rene Caisse died in 1978 at the age of ninety. She spent a frustrating life trying to save people's lives with a simple herbal tea, only to have that effort thwarted by the politics and greed of the medical establishment. Not much has changed since.

CHAPTER TWO

Testimonials

"Testimonials are

important pieces of evidence...

they are testimony to

the human capacity for healing."

Andrew Weil, M.D.

*T*hese testimonials represent the recent experience of a few people with Essiac and should not be taken as suggestions for treatment.

"Four years ago I was in my early forties and diagnosed with lymphoma. The doctors administered chemotherapy for four months. They told me that my cancer had spread to my organs, liver and spleen. For the next year the tests showed no improvement and lumps began to appear under my chin. Shortly after that I started on Essiac super blue-green algae. I take two ounces of the Essiac three times daily. At night I mix the Essiac with distilled water and drink it like a tea. The doses of chemotherapy made me so ill, I would throw up and my weight went down to seventy-nine pounds. I have been off chemotherapy for three years now. I did have the lymph nodes removed from my right side. I haven't had a cold in four years. I was at death's door and today I am running."

S.M.

"My wife has been taking Essiac for almost two years now along with several other non-traditional treatments. My wife has low-grade mixed cell lymphoma in fourth stage. She is alive and well today."

J.M.

"I lost my mother a year ago to breast cancer. She was two months short of 104 and the treatment was directed towards maintaining a good quality of life as long as possible. Essiac was a part of that treatment and she certainly did a lot better than the doctors expected."

D.F.

"My husband began using Essiac one week after discovering the tumor. He has multiple myeloma. We are eating much more home-grown foods, less meat, and many more vegetables. He also takes many multiple vitamins per day as well as the powdered juice of green barley. He cut back on caffeine, junk food, and canned goods. My husband takes four ounces of Essiac a day: two in the morning and two at night before bed. At first nothing seemed to be happening. He did note, however, that he felt stronger and had more energy. If he missed a day he could really feel it the next day. The cancer in fact got much worse before it improved. He is on a very potent chemotherapy drug (cytoxin), yet he has had no hair loss, no nausea, no tiredness, no pain, and no more bone deterioration. The doctors are surprised and impressed at his progress. He is surpassing all their expectations."

> **"The doctors are surprised and impressed at his progress. He has surpassed all their expectations."**

M.S.

"I have been using Essiac for both myself and clients for 4 years and have found that it not only has positive results with some cancers, but also as an overall detoxifier tonic for other conditions, to maintain health, stimulate immune responses and prevent illnesses. It seems to help the body eliminate toxic metals as well."

K.W.

"I have breast cancer that was diagnosed in February of 1994. I had two partial mastectomies followed by chemo, then radiation. I began taking the Essiac in May. In July I had a bone scan and liver MRI and they didn't find any cancer in either of these tests. I am taking the Essiac to prevent a recurrence. I have chosen not to take tomoxifen because I don't want any more chemicals in my body. I am trying to rebuild my immune system so that my body can fight off any remaining cancer. Essiac had been suggested to me after my first surgery, but I decided to go the conventional route and opted for chemotherapy and radiation. When I realized that was not totally effective, I began looking for alternatives. One of these alternatives(along with acupuncture and heavy doses of Vitamin E) is Essiac."

J.H.

"In August of 1993, I was diagnosed with chronic, late stage hepatitis "C." I was constantly fatigued and suffering chronic pain in the liver region. I lost 30 pounds and my eyes were dull and sunken back into my head. The doctors knew how to treat hepatitis "A" and "B," but knew very little about "C." They tried experimental drugs that were of little success. They told me my only alternative was a liver transplant.

"A friend suggested I try Essiac tea. I tried it and noticed an immediate reduction of pain. As I continued to take Essiac, I began to regain my weight and felt less depressed. My pain did not disappear, but was reduced 90%, and my health improved overall with lab results to prove it. I still have the virus, but my immune system is stronger, which gives me a quality of life I would not have had if I hadn't tried Essiac."

R.M.

"Twelve years ago, Michelle Kalevik of Denver was diagnosed by the allopathic medical community as having an "incurable disease." The doctors wanted to perform radical surgery. Michelle shares, "At that point, I chose to empower myself by choosing alternative health and healing on all levels of the mind-body connection. After using *Ojibwa Tea of Life* formula, I am alive and well twelve years later. I encourage others to follow their heart, and to pursue the myriad of holistic health modalities that are available to us. The ` healing' journey can be one of the most enlightening experiences of our lives."

Michelle is a Reiki practitioner
and the founder of a support group
for people whoare HIV positive.
She is a supplier of an Essiac product
called Ojibwa Tea of Life. Her address
can be found in the Resources section.

Charles A. Brusch, MD
15 Grozier Rd.
Cambridge, Massachusetts 02138

April 6, 1990

TO WHOM IT MAY CONCERN:
Many years have gone by since I first experienced the use of ESSIAC with my patients who were suffering from many varied forms of cancer.

I personally monitored the use of this old therapy along with Rene Caisse, R.N., whose many successes were widely reported. Rene worked with me at my medical clinic in Cambridge, Massachusetts and where, under the supervision of 18 of my many medical doctors on staff, she proceeded with a series of treatments on terminal cancer patients and laboratory mice and together we refined and perfected her formula.

On mice it has been shown to cause a decided recession of the mass and a definite change in cell formation.

Clinically, on patients suffering from pathologically proven cancer, it reduces pain and causes a recession in the growth. Patients gained weight and showed a great improvement in their general health. Their elimination improved considerably and their appetite became whetted.

> **"Remarkable beneficial results were obtained even on those cases at the 'end of the road' where it proved to prolong life and the 'quality' of that life."**

Remarkable beneficial results were obtained even on those cases at the "end of the road" where it proved to prolong life and the "quality" of that life.

In some cases, if the tumor didn't disappear, it could be surgically removed after ESSIAC with less risk of metastases resulting in new outbreaks.

Hemorrhage has been rapidly brought under control in many difficult cases, open lesions of lip and breast responded to treatment, and patients with cancer of the stomach have returned to normal activity among many other remembered cases. Also, intestinal burns from radiation were healed and damage replaced, and it was found to greatly improve whatever the condition.

All these patients' cases were diagnosed by reputable physicians and surgeons.

I do know that I have witnessed in my clinic and know of many other cases where ESSIAC was the therapy used, a treatment which brings about restoration through destroying the tumor tissue and improving the mental outlook which re-establishes physiological function.

> **"I endorse this therapy even today for I have in fact cured my own cancer, the original site of which was the lower bowel, through ESSIAC alone."**

I endorse this therapy even today for I have in fact cured my own cancer, the original site of which was the lower bowel, through ESSIAC alone.

In my last complete examination, where I was examined throughout the intestinal tract while hospitalized (August, 1989) for a hernia problem, no sign of malignancy was found. Medical documents validate this.

I have taken ESSIAC every day since my diagnosis (1984) and my recent examination has given me a clear bill of health.

I remained a partner with Rene Caisse until her death in 1978 and was the only person who had her complete trust and to whom she confided her knowledge and "know-how" of what she named "ESSIAC."

Others have imitated, but a minor success rate should never be accepted when the true therapy is available.

Rene Caisse R.N. & Dr. Brusch M.D., Clinical Records and Observations

Often patients would report an enlarging and hardening of the tumor after a few treatments, then the tumor would begin to soften, and if it was located in any body system with a route to the exterior, the patient would report discharging large amounts of pus and fleshy material. After this, she said, the tumor would be gone.

> **"Rene felt that Essiac caused all the cancerous cells to retreat to the site of the original tumor. Then to shrink and discharge — often to vanish altogether."**

Rene felt that Essiac caused all the cancerous cells to retreat to the site of the original tumor. Then to shrink and discharge—often to vanish altogether.

In some cases she found that if

the tumor didn't disappear, it could be surgically removed after Essiac with less risk of metastases (or spreading) resulting in new outbreaks.

"I achieved good results in animal research, under the observation of medical doctors. My treatments caused a regression of the malignant growth in the mice, and prolonged life." Rene Caisse.

She believed that radium treatment actually drives cancer farther into the body and burns the tissue which creates more cancer. Essiac can strengthen the body and if the cancer is localized, surgery can remove the cancerous lesion without disturbing recurrence.

In breast cancer cases, Rene felt that both breasts would eventually be affected with cancer. If Essiac injections were given in the forearm, the secondary mass would regress, enlarging the primary mass for a time until it could localize, soften and become easier to remove.

Cancer of the lung: Rene stated she advised treatment with Essiac before removal of the lung.

If surgery is required, six or eight treatments of Essiac may make surgery more successful. After surgery, Essiac should be taken once a week for at least three months.

CHAPTER THREE

Herbs and Healing

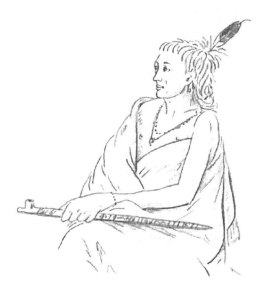

To the Great Spirit

Your Spirit,

my spirit,

may they unite in healing.

You have given your beauty,

now we ask that you give

the gift of well being.

Ojibwa Healing Song

$\mathcal{H}$erbs not only continue to abundantly feed us, but until the beginning of the last century they served as our principal healing vehicle, and still do in many cultures around the world. Modern herb-alists and traditional healers alike hold that there is an herb or herbal combination for every malady known to man. Prior to the gradual development of chemical and biochemical methods during the 18th and 19th centuries, herbalism was an integral part of western medicine. Hippocrates, often called the father of western medicine, used about 400 drugs, most of which were of herbal ori-gin. The development of science and the scientific method helped spell the end of herbalism as an important part of modern medicine. It came to be considered old fashioned, superstitious, or second class.

The growth of the highly profitable pharmaceutical industry, beginning in the early 20th century, put the final seal on the separation of mainstream medicine and traditional herbalism. Prior to that time there were still a fair number of physicians who carefully integrated local herbal lore, including that of the Native Americans, into their practice.

THE NATIVE HEALER

A medicine man or woman is often the spiritual leader of the community. She or he will typically train under a mentor for many years to assimilate countless generations of accumulated knowledge and wisdom. This includes spiritual lore as well as the identification and use of the local medicinal herbs. Healing practice usually involves ceremony, and sometimes the use of the sweat lodge, along with medicinal herbs.

Native healers or shamans are often also shrewd psychologists who understand the power of the mind and the effect of emotional energy in creating and dispelling disease. They understand how important the beliefs of the patient are in the healing process. Spiritual guidance and intuition also play an important part in traditional native healing.

The Midewiwin Medicine Society of the Ojibwa

The "old Indian medicine man" who introduced the herbal formula to the woman who gave it in turn thirty years later to Rene Caisse, could well have been a member of the Midewiwin, the Grand Medicine Society of the Ojibwa. Loosely translated, Midewiwin means: "things done to the sounds of the drum."

The Ojibwa derived from a people who called themselves the Anishinabe, the Original People, who had lived on the Atlantic coast of Canada. The Anishinabe migrated inland after being warned "If you do not move, you will be destroyed," by a prophet who may have been predicting the coming of the white man. Visions that were promised by the prophet eventually led them to the Great Lakes where they split into three groups. Each group accepted a different responsibility for sustaining the culture.

The Potawatomi, who ended up on the eastern shore of Lake Michigan, pledged to safeguard the sacred fire. The Ottawa, who settled on Manitoulin Island in Lake Huron, agreed to become traders. The third group, the Ojibwa, would preserve the sacred lore of the people in words, in songs, and in symbols inscribed on birch-bark scrolls. The Midewiwin was formed for this purpose.

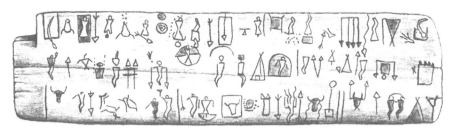

Ojibwa Song Inscribed on the Lid of a Midewiwin's Medicine Box

The Ojibwa, who settled on the northern shore of Lake Superior, were the least affected by the encroaching Europeans. The densely wooded terrain not only afforded protection but was unattractive to farmers. They were largely left in peace and were even able to expand their territory into what is now Minnesota and central Ontario. With over 200,000 members today, the Ojibwa represent one of North America's largest native groups.

The activities of the Midewiwin also evolved and expanded over time. The society's ceremonies grew increasingly complex, combining the tribe's creation myth, the vision quest, and herbal medicine. A structured system was developed for training new members in the various ceremonies and healing procedures as well as the use of medicinal herbs. It has been said that the tribes around the Great Lakes were familiar with as many as 400 plants for treating illness.

> **"It has been said that the tribes around the Great Lakes were familiar with as many as 400 plants for treating illness."**

A Great Medicine Dance was held each spring and sometimes in the fall. This was primarily an initiation ceremony for new Midewiwin members. Each student was selected by a tutor (elder Mide) for a one-year period of instruction. The student must be selected anew each year by his or her mentor. The initiation ceremony included the symbolic death and rebirth of each candidate. The initiates each received a beaver skin medicine bag that contained sacred objects as well as medicinal herbs.

The course of study lasted for four, and sometimes even eight years. A fee was paid to the tutor that was quite affordable at first but that increased with each year. This was probably to ensure the commitment of the student. As in other Native American cultures, the vision quest is a central part of an individual Ojibwa's spiritual experience. This is especially true for a practicing Mide. Combining fasting and thirsting with a solitary wilderness retreat, the vision quest involves a visionary relationship with a totem animal that characterizes the nature of the individual's spirit helpers. The "medicine" or power manifested by this relationship sets the tone for that individual's speciality or unique approach to healing. An individual pursues the first vision quest at about the time of puberty and repeats the experience as needed in later years.

The Midewiwin still thrives today and fits right in with the recent revival of interest in holistic, alternative healing practices, including herbalism. While something like a quarter of modern pharmaceutical medicines are still extracted from plant materials, more and more people are realizing that the original whole plant with all its minute ingredients, is the complete remedy - Nature's perfect gift. The search for safe, natural remedies is particularly intense in the field of cancer treatment, where mainstream medical techniques such as surgery, radiation and chemotherapy are not only expensive, but often seem as destructive as the disease itself. Many today are seeking milder, yet effective, alternatives. Rene Caisse, with her successful use of Essiac, was a pioneer in this movement.

First Year Midewiwin Initiate's Medicine Bag

CHAPTER FOUR

The Essiac Herbs

"And God said, behold,

I have given you every herb bearing seed...

let it serve as food."

Genesis 1:29

*A*ll four of the ingredients in Essiac have been used as food in various cultures.

BURDOCK

Botanical Name: Arctium lappa, A. minus

Common Names: Beggar's buttons, clotbur, cocklebur, hardock, turkey burseed, burr seed, gobo root

Medicinal Part: The root is used for Essiac. Stems, flowers, seeds, and occasionally leaves, are also used medicinally.

Description: Burdock is a biennial plant described as a troublesome weed found growing throughout southern Canada and the United States, where it was brought from

45

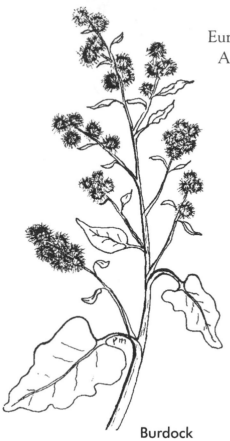

Burdock

Europe by early settlers, as well as Asia and Japan.

The herb has long dull green stalks of up to twelve inches in height. The oval leaves have many veins; the underside has a fine gray down appearance while the leaves and stalk have purple patterns. In the second year of growth the plant produces purple blossoms which grow up to three feet tall. Burdock, a close relative to echinacea and dandelion, is sought after for its healing properties as well as the culinary uses of the young greens and stalk. Harvest the long, fleshy gray root in the fall of the first year or the spring of the second year.

Therapeutic Action:

Burdock is regarded as an immune system strengthener, a tonic for the liver, kidneys and lungs as well as a blood purifier with the ability to neutralize poisons and cleanse the lymphatic system. Burdock contains proven anti-bacterial and anti-fungal as well as tumor-protective compounds. The leaves contain a substance which promotes bile secretion and may be included in liver and gall bladder formulas. An infusion or decoction of the root may be used as a skin wash for burns, ringworm, acne and rashes. A poultice using the leaf material will treat gout.

In the Orient, burdock root is used for its nutritive and strengthening qualities. In Hawaii it is known by the Japanese name Gobo root' and is used to increase strength and endurance. In China, where the seed pod is dried and used for coughs, colds, measles, boils and sore throats, burdock has been found listed as a useful medicine as early as 502 AD. It is also noted as medicinal by Cherokees, Menomonee and Micmac Native Americans who used it for skin sores.

Vitamin & Mineral Content: Calcium (50mg), phosphorus (58mg), iron (1.2mg), sodium (30mg), thiamine (0.25mg.), riboflavin (.88 mg.), niacin (0.3mg), Vitamin C (2mg)

Preparation and Dosage: One ounce of burdock root makes one quart of tea.

Precautions: Burdock may have estrogen-like effects and therefore should be avoided during pregnancy.

SHEEP SORREL

Botanical Name: Acetosella vulgaris [formerly Rumex Acetosella Polygonaceae]

Common Name: Dog-eared sorrel, field sorrel, red top sorrel

Medicinal Part: Whole plant, leaves.

Description: Sheep Sorrel is a perennial plant that grows in rocky areas throughout the world with the exception of the tropics. The plant is common along roadsides in England and is sometimes cultivated in the United States. The whole plant can be used before the stem is hollow in the second year. The roots are woody, long and tapering. The furrowed or streaked stem grows one to two feet high. The edible leaves are attached to the stem by a slender leaf stalk and are green, the pigment indicating a high amount of Chlorophyll.

Leaves are ovate with two lateral teeth. Upper part is oblong and narrow. Green flowers with reddish tinge distinguish from the oranage-red female flowers. Sheep sorrel seeds are shiny, black, three-sided small seeds resembling peppercorn.

Sheep Sorrel

Harvest the plant early in the day or in late afternoon May through August before it flowers and goes to seed in September.

Therapeutic Action:

The whole herb when young and in its freshest state acts as a diuretic and blood cleanser. The herb improves liver, intestinal and bowel functions, prevents destruction of red blood cells and is used to break down tumors. The chlorophyll in sheep sorrel leaves carries oxygen through the bloodstream which strengthens cell walls, helps remove deposits in blood vessels and allows the body to store and use more oxygen. Chlorophyll may also reduce radiation damage and restrict chromosome damage. The herb is smooth and acid while the root has astringent properties and contains a substance allied to crysophanic acid (an iron-greening tannin diuretic). Sheep sorrel is taken for inflammatory diseases, tumors, incipient cancers and urine and kidney diseases. The action is refrigerant, diaphoretic and diuretic.

Preparation and Dosage:

One bushel fresh herb yields one pound powder.

TURKEY RHUBARB

Botanical Name: Rheum palmatum

Common Names: Chinese rhubarb, East India rhubarb

Medicinal Part: Root stock of older plants without the periderm.

Description: Turkey Rhubarb somewhat resembles the garden variety rhubarb (rheum rhaponticum) but medicinally is quite a bit stronger. A perennial, the herb is identified by its conical, fleshy root stock with yellow interior. The seven-lobed, heart shaped or rounded leaves grow twelve to eighteen inches in length and are attached by thick petioles to stems five to ten feet tall. Topping the hollow flower stem is a leafy panicle of greenish or whitish flowers. Turkey rhubarb is cultivated in China and Tibet for decorative as well as medicinal purposes.

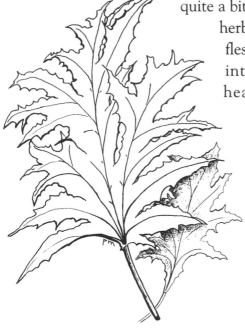

Turkey Rhubarb

Therapeutic Actions: Turkey rhubarb has been used for centuries for its dual action as a laxative and astringent as well as a purging treatment. In smaller doses it is used to treat diarrhea or to stimulate the appetite. Larger amounts yield a laxative effect. The herb stimulates the colon and abates distension while promoting bile flow, clearing stasis and restoring the stomach and liver. It has been used as a stomach tonic to soothe digestion; to cleanse the liver; as an anti-tumor; and an aid for thermal burns, jaundice, sores and cancers. As a regulator, turkey rhubarb has both contractive and dilative properties that help regulate menstruation and eliminative processes. It is versatile in preparations as a balancing herb and anthelmintic.

In Chinese medicine, its properties are considered bitter and cold entering the stomach, colon, liver, spleen and pericardium meridians. Functions to drain heat and dampness, moves stools, cools blood, disperses and invigorates stagnant blood.

Preparation and Dosage: Soak the root stock in cold water to make a cold extract or use chopped, powdered dry herb or tincture.

For a calming and astringent effect: 1/4 tsp powdered or six drops tincture every 60 minutes.

For a gastrointestinal stasis or as a laxative: 1 tsp powdered, 1/4-1/2 tbsp tincture, or 1 tbl cold extract liquid.

Precautions: The leaf blades are very poisonous, causing vomiting and liver and kidney damage. The herb contains oxalic acid and pro longed or exaggerated use during preg nancy or lactation should be avoided.

SLIPPERY ELM

Botanical Name: Ulmus fulva

Common Names: Red elm, moose elm, Indian elm

Medicinal Part: Inner bark

Description: Slippery elm can be found in northern and central United States and eastern Canada. It grows in moist woods and bottom land, along streams, as well as in dry soil. The rough branches and long, tough, hairy leaves help distinguish slippery elm which re- sembles a small tree and can grow up to sixty feet tall.

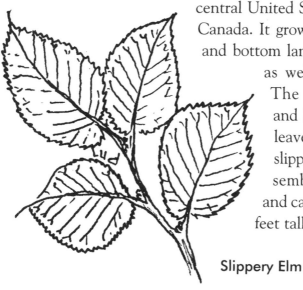

Slippery Elm

The dark green or yellowish leaves are covered with yellow wool and have orange tips, while the bark is deeply furrowed. The pinkish white, fibrous inner bark contains the healing properties. The inner bark can be obtained whole or powdered. In its powdered state it is pale pink brown in color.

Therapeutic Actions:

Slippery elm is good for nervous problems, stomach and intestines, sore throats and coughs. It contains inulin which helps liver, spleen and pancreas. The herb promotes urination, disperses swelling and acts as a laxative. Chinese medicine listed the herb in 25 BC and noted that it is good for diarrhea, ulcers, soothing inflamed colon, small intestine, and colon meridians. It has a sweet flavor with a neutral property. Indians used it as a demulcent, salve and laxative. Some believe it may help diabetic conditions.

Preparation and Dosage:

Peel the bark from older trees when the sap is still running. Pull the juicy quarter-inch-thick inner bark away in long strips and let dry. The powdered bark can be mixed with hot milk or water and made into a nutritious breakfast meal or a relaxing nighttime drink.

Slippery elm can be prepared as a bolus, or suppository-shaped poultice, for internal use: Heat cocoa butter over hot water, stir in slippery elm. Allow to cool and roll into several boluses the width of middle finger cut into one-inch lengths. When they have hardened, insert vaginally followed by a tampon which will control the melting that will occur. It works on the GI tract soothing inflamed colon and is a good nutrient when food cannot be kept down. Use in a poultice form to treat burns, respiratory infections, fevers, wounds, boils, skin infections.

Precautions: No toxicity for internal or external use found.

CHAPTER FIVE

The Essiac Formula

"Anyone who doesn't

believe in miracles

is not a realist."

David Ben-Gurion

ESSIAC TEA FORMULA AND DIRECTIONS

Dry Ingredients

Burdock Root (cut)   6.5 cups (52 measuring cup ounces)

Sheep Sorrel (powder)   16.0 ounces (scale weight)

Slippery Elm Bark (powder) 4.0 ounces (scale wieight)

Turkey Rhubarb Root (")   1.0 ounces (scale weight)

Wet Ingredients

Distilled, sodium-free distilled, spring, or thoroughly filtered water

Ingredients' Yields

8 measuring cup ounces of dry ingredients plus 2 gallons of water yields around 224 liquid ounces (fourteen 16-ounce bottles) of tea.

4 measuring cup ounces of dry ingredients plus 1 gallon of water yields around 112 liquid ounces (seven 16-ounce bottles) of tea.

2 measuring cup ounces of dry ingredients and 0.5 gal-lons of water yields around 56 liquid ounces (three and one-half 16-ounce bottles) of tea.

Supplies Needed

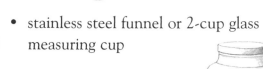

• two glass or stainless steel pots (one with lid)

• stainless steel fine mesh strainer

• large stainless steel or wood stirring utensil

• stainless steel funnel or 2-cup glass measuring cup

• storage containers: dark amber glass bottles with air tight caps or mason jars with air tight lids

Note 1: The sizes of the pots and the number or size of storage containers depends on the amount of tea prepared.

Note 2: Storage containers must be sterilized. Steriliza-tion options (principally for glass bottles and caps):

a) Boil for 10 minutes with a little food grade peroxide or Clorox.

b) Boil bottle caps: put bottles in 250 degree oven for 10 minutes.

c) Soak for 5 minutes in 1 ounce 35% food grade hydro-gen peroxide and 11 ounces distilled water.

d) Soak for 5 minutes in 1/2 teaspoon Clorox and 1 gallon distilled water.

Preparation

1. Mix dry ingredients thoroughly.

2. Measure out desired amount of dry ingredients. (Store remainder in cool, dark place as ingredients are light sensitive.)

3. Pour proportionate amount of water into pot.

4. Bring water to a rolling boil with the lid on.

5. Stir dry ingredients into boiling water.

6. Replace lid and continue boiling at reduced heat for 10 minutes.

7. Turn off stove. Scrape down sides of pot and stir mix-ture thoroughly.

8. Replace lid and allow pot to sit and cool for 6 hours.

9. Stir thoroughly. Replace lid and let mixture sit for another 6 hours.

Note: It is acceptable to skip this step and let mixture sit undisturbed for 12 hours.

10. Return mixture to burner and reheat to the boiling point, but do not boil.

11. Turn off heat and strain contents into second pot.

12. Clean first pot and strainer.

13. Strain contents back into first pot.

14. Immediately pour hot liquid into sterilized storage containers.

15. Allow storage containers to cool, then tighten tops.

16. Refrigerate.

Note 1: Essiac contains no preservative agents.

Note 2: If mold should develop, discard immediately.

Note 3: An argument can be made for refrigerating a storage container only when it has been opened, storing the remainder in a cool, dark cupboard.

DIRECTIONS FOR USE AS A PREVENTATIVE

- Take at bedtime on an empty stomach (at least two hours after eating): 4 tablespoons (2 ounces), warm or cold.

- Tea can be taken in the morning: take before eating and do not eat for two hours.

- Tea can also be diluted with equal parts of water.

- Before pouring tea from container, shake gently to mix any sediment that has settled.

- Do not microwave.

Directions for Use

- Take 2 ounces twice a day, two hours before or after eating. Ideally, take in the morning on an empty stomach and wait two hours before eating, and take at bedtime, two hours after eating. Tea can also be diluted with equal parts of water.
- Before pouring tea from container, shake gently to mix any sediment that has settled.
- Do not microwave.

Notes on Use

- If stomach cancer, dilute with equal parts of water.
- Though side affects are rare when taking Essiac, there are three general ones:

1) nausea and/or indigestion, generally caused by eating or drinking too soon before or after drinking the tea,

2) severe intestinal or digestive discomfort, caused principally because as toxins dissolve, the body tries to eliminate them quickly,

3) an increase in the size of an existing tumor, caused by the metastasized cells gathering at the original site, before the tumor softens and reduces in size.

If discomfort occurs, stop taking the tea for several days until feeling better. Then begin taking it again in half-ounce doses every other day, and gradually increase the interval and dosage to the desired levels.

OTHER HERBS THAT MAY BE ADDED

Dandelion root has the capacity to clear obstruction and stimulate the liver to detoxify poisons. Clears obstruction of the spleen, pancreas, gallbladder, bladder and kidney. I consider it a specific for high blood pressure, hypoglycemia, elevated blood lipids, sodium retention, elimination of uric acid and diabetes. It is a blood purifier with high, easily assailable mineral content. Good for those individuals with a diet high in poor quality fats and proteins with a tendency toward arteriosclerosis (males) and gallstone (females).

Mullein flowers for respiratory ailments, as an expectorant and demulcent for the lungs, urinary irritability, diuretic, lymphatic congestion and as a nervine, astringent and antispasmodic

Fenugreek seeds as a tonic, astringent, demulcent, emollient and expectorant. Useful for all mucus conditions and lung congestion. It helps eliminate excess mucus, is useful for ulcers and inflamed conditions of the stomach and intestines. Is used as a treatment for both gout and diabetes. I consider it a rejuvenator for the digestion.

Red root for its ability to strengthen intestinal tissues, improves the positive charge of the blood, strengthens bogginess of the lymph pulp and nodes. It helps increase the efficiency of transport of nutrients from the blood across the capillary cells to the lymph and increased efficiency of lymph transport of waste products, away from the cells and eventually back to the blood and liver. It prevents the buildup of congested fluids in the lymphatic tissue. For breast cysts, fluid cysts, ovarian cysts, testicular hydroceles, tonsil and sinus inflammations, sore throats, enlarged lymph nodes, enlarged spleen, menstrual hemorrhage, nosebleeds, hemorrhoids, and old ulcers.

Ocotillo for pelvic fluid congestion, both lymphatic and veinous, poor fluid movement and congestion in the lower viscera and pelvis. Improves dietary fat absorption into the lymph system. Helps hemorrhoids, cervical varicosites and benign prostate enlargements. Frequent need to urinate, with dull ache but no inflammation of the urethra, varicose veins and piles worsened by constipation or poor digestion.

Contributed by Kendra Whittaker, Clinical Herbalist

CHAPTER SIX

Cancer and Lifestyle

"Mind is the master power

that moulds and makes, and man is mind,

and evermore he takes the tool of thought,

and shaping what he wills,

brings forth a thousand joys, a thousand ills."

James Allen

*A*ccording to physician Bernie Siegel, only 15 to 20% of people with chronic or catastrophic illness can be called survivors. In other words, they are willing to take responsibility for their condition, redirect their lives, and participate in their own recovery. The majority, 50-60%, are content to sit back and let their doctors direct their treatment ("You're the doctor, fix me!"). The remaining 20% are secretly happy to die because their life is in a shambles.

A healthy lifestyle can be quite simply described, and you've no doubt heard much of it before. It may not be so easy to do: Love yourself. Keep fit. Move and stretch regularly in a way that feels right for you. Eat the right foods in moderation. Love yourself. Avoid that which is possibly harmful. Stay focused in the present and think positive, peaceful thoughts. Learn to acknowledge and express *all* your emotions and quickly release them. Love yourself.

Laugh a lot. Cultivate and honor your intuition. Give yourself the gift of regular solitude, preferably in a natural environment. Be honest—especially with yourself. Love yourself. Reduce stress through a practice of regular meditation, intentional loving, allowing and detachment. Reconnect with your Creator, your higher self, by consciously cultivating faith, hope, trust, and surrender. Learn to live with reverence and gratitude. But most of all, love yourself!

"Learn to live with reverence and gratitude. But most of all, love yourself!"

And if none of this works, maybe it's simply time to complete this physical phase of a journey that is essentially spiritual, and move on. So be it. Let it be and let go. Nearly all who have sampled the experience—who have gone and come back—say it's wonderful. And if you don't believe it, read the works of those who have written about the near death experience such as Drs. Elizabeth Kubler-Ross, Raymond Moody, Kenneth Ring and others.

THE MIND/BODY CONNECTION

Doctors have long acknowledged the influence our thought patterns have on the body, but usually only among themselves. Freshman medical texts sometimes admit that as much as 50% of dis-ease is psychosomatic, in other words, "of the mind." For physicians to admit that much of disease is rooted in the mind would put them out of business, leaving only the psychiatrists to practice medicine!

Recently though, we are hearing a few forthright M.D.s actually speak publicly about the effect of one's thoughts upon the physical body. The eloquent and increasingly popular Deepak Chopra tells how an individual thought can instantly impact the body via the creation of a neurotransmitter or hormone.

An Arizona physician, Robert Koppen, M.D., has written: "Thought, combined with feeling, generates a strong creative energy that will not fail to bring about results in the physical world; and whether or not the one who has these thoughts and feelings believes this to be true makes no difference."

Dr. Koppen goes on to say that ". . .the body mind connection is a two edged sword. If we are in a happy, contented, peaceful state of mind, and appreciate the beauty of nature as an expression of Divine intelligence and love, then our thoughts and feelings will amplify the beauty of our world and the health of our body that can be enjoyed. But if we are unhappy, angry, blaming the world, ourselves or God for our self-generated and perpetuated misery, then the physical results of our inner attitude can become quite destructive to our mental, emotional and physical health."

Emotions and Cancer

While our mental experience can have a very real and direct influence upon our bodies and thus, our health, our emotional experience may have an even greater impact in the long run. An emotion is typically a habitual response to unconscious mental activity. Our unconscious thoughts are the result of our perceptions and the way we assume the world works. All this is founded upon who we basically are along with our subconscious belief system which was largely in place at a very early age. We are still dealing with the mind/body connection but with emotions as an intermediate process. Emotions are a very real form of energy that can have a substantial impact on the body and its health.

> **"When it comes to cancer, however, the problem seems to be not so much in experiencing negative emotions as in not experiencing them or not wanting to experience them."**

When it comes to cancer, however, the problem seems to be not so much in experiencing negative emotions as in *not* experiencing them or not *wanting* to experience them. Dr. Marjorie Brooks, of Jefferson Medical College in Philadelphia, discovered that women who were very, very seldom angry along with women who were highly volatile were more likely to have malignant tumors than women who had an appropriate expression of anger. She also learned that women with malignant breast cancer were more likely to apologize for their anger, even when they were right. And when they did express their hostility, they often took it back. Women who tended to get angry and stay angry were also subject to tumors but not as frequently as those who didn't express at all. Women in normal health were more likely to get angry and let it go.

Psychologist Dennis Jaffe, PhD, says that "The cancer pattern is well established in the literature. It's characterized by feelings of helplessness and hopelessness — the feeling that you've been victimized by factors beyond your control that you have no power to change. The healthy person seems to actively take care of the things that need to be taken care of and has the capacity to say 'no, that's not my problem, I'm not going to waste my energy worrying about things beyond my control.' She has a sense of personal power—not over powered or underpowered."

In a long-term study, Dr. Richard B. Shekelle of the University of Texas School of Medicine followed the lives of 2000 men. Those who scored highest in the tests for depression died twice as often of cancer as the others. Caroline B. Thomas, M.D., of the Johns Hopkins School of Medicine, discovered that cancer patients often had a prior poor ("neither admiring or comfortable") relationship with their parents.

Understanding why one feels a certain way can no doubt help resolve negative emotions but the real message is clear: acknowledge them, have them, let them go.

CANCER AND NUTRITION

In 1988, the Surgeon General stated that a reduction of fat in the diet could help prevent cancer as well as other chronic diseases. Organically grown foods are free from potentially carcinogenic pesticides and chemical additives. They also are richer in health giving nutrients including beta carotene, vitamin E and selenium. Daily doses of these three nutrients can reduce cancer deaths up to 13%. It may be advisable to consult with your health practitioner on suggested dosages of any of the supplements listed here.

Live Enzymes

Enzymes have been found to be vitally important for digestion and immune system functioning. With age, enzyme production tends to decrease and so illness increases. There are three classifications of enzymes: digestive, food and metabolic.

Digestive enzymes: If these are lacking, our bodies cannot digest the foods we eat. Not only are essential nutrients lost, but the resulting putrification and decay produces harmful toxins.

Food enzymes: Raw foods also contain enzymes that aid digestion. When food is cooked over 120 degrees, most enzymes are destroyed. Cooked foods can also over stress organs and cause deterioration.

Metabolic enzymes: White blood cells (leukocytes) contain protease (protein digestive enzymes), amylase (starch digestive enzymes) and lipase {fat digestive enzymes). White blood cells attack alien substances. The combination of eating raw foods and taking supplements will aid the white blood cells in keeping the immune system and blood healthy. Taking supplements only at meal time helps ensure that vitamins and supplements will be fully utilized by the body.

Cancer Fighting Foods

Beta-carotene: Found in most leafy green vegetables, sweet potatoes, carrots and spinach. Good as a preventative for cervical, stomach, lung, and oral cancer. Suggested dosage: 25,000 IU.

Vitamin B6: (pyridoxine) Found in sweet potatoes, carrots, organ meats, leafy green vegetables, bananas and apples. For cervical cancer, healthy mucus membranes, immune function, Suggested dosage: up to 1,000 mg per day.

Vitamin C: (calcium ascorbate) Citrus fruits, vegetables, broccoli, green peppers. Helps sustain healthy immune system. Suggested dosage: 50-10,000 mg daily.

Vitamin E: (mixed tocopherols) Unrefined vegetable oils, wheat germ, leafy green vegetables, and various herbs. Supreme antioxidant bowel, breast, and lung cancer. Suggested dosage: 100-1,000 mg daily with meals.

Calcium: Found in dark green vegetables, sardines and salmon, as well as many seeds and nuts. Promotes cell metabolism, blood clotting, along with healthy bones and teeth. May be helpful for colon cancer. Suggested dosage: 1,000-1,500 mg per day.

Zinc: (gluconates, picolinates) Soybeans, sunflower seeds, seafoods, onions, whole grains, garbanzos, lentils, peas. Promotes rna/dna production, immune function. Suggested for prostate cancer. Suggested dosage: 20-100 mg per day.

Garlic: Preventative in general. May inhibit tumor growth.

Folic Acid: Fish, citrus fruits, cabbage, beets, eggs, dark green leafy vegetables. May be helpful for cervical cancer. Promotes rna/dna synthesis. Suggested daily dose: 400-2,000 mcg.

Iodine: Seafood, sea vegetables. Preventative for breast cancer. Promotes tissue growth and repair. Suggested daily dose: 100-1000 mcg.

Omega-3 Fatty Acids: Salmon, sardines, haddock, cod. Preventive for breast cancer; aids tissue and cell function.

Omega-6 Fatty Acids: Evening primrose oil. Suggested dosage: one tablespoon daily.

Magnesium: Brown rice, nuts, whole grains, green vegetables. Assists rna/dna synthesis, ph of tissue and blood. General cancer preventative. Suggested daily dose: 300-800 mg.

Lactobacillius Acidophilus: Capsule, powder, live yogurt cultures. May help prevent colon cancer.

Iodine: For breast, endometrial and ovarian cancer. Suggested daily dose: 100-1,000 mcg.

Selenium: A trace mineral, is found in fruits and vegetables. It is an antioxidant and aids the body in producing glutathione, an enzyme that aids detoxification. Daily dosage: 200-300 mcg. Wait half an hour before taking vitamin C.

Parasite Cleansing: Statistics reveal that, according to the World Health Organization, 16.4 million people died in 1993 of parasites and infectious diseases. In 1994 that figure rose to 1.5 billion. An individual can come into contact with parasites through contaminated food, water, undercooked meat, fish, unsanitary conditions, and from pets. Children are more apt to come into contact with parasites because of the amount of time spent playing outside. Today, over 500 million children are infected with parasites.

Cancer and parasites are closely linked. We have stressed that a consumption of healthy, live food is important, and that over-processed foods such as junk food, sugar and hydrogenated oils create an environment where parasites flourish. This environment, caused by poor diet, allows parasites to feed upon, and eventually to starve the body of all nutrients, thus resulting in disease.

There exist over 100 different types of parasites. Symptoms of infection include bloating, fatigue. diarrhea, anemia, low blood sugar, runny nose, headaches, hair loss, teeth grinding and mineral imbalances. There are several treatments to rid the body of parasites which may take anywhere from three weeks to three months to accomplish. A combination of black walnut hulls (black walnut tree) and wormwood (Artemesia shrub) kills 100 types of parasites in the developmental stage, and cloves {clove tree) kills the eggs.

A formula by Hanna Kroeger contains pumpkin seeds, capsium, thyme, garlic, and cramp bark. Since parasites don't survive well in an acidic environment, one may also increase acidic foods such as cranberry juice, apple cider vinegar, garlic, figs, or pumpkin seeds. Sources for these products can be found listed in the resource directory at the end of the book.

Foods to Avoid or Greatly Moderate

Caffeine, coffee, tea, chocolate, soft drinks: Associated with bladder and urinary tract cancer, as well as rna/dna damage.

Refined sugar and eggs: Have been connected with ovarian cancer.

Fried foods; partially hydrogenated oils; salt; cured and pickled foods; saccharin, cyclamates, butylated hydroxytouluene; fried, barbecued and broiled meats; fish and chicken cooked at high temperatures; milk, peanuts, corn: Contain aflatoxins and have been associated with kidney, liver and stomach cancer.

Dairy products: Contain growth hormones which may contribute to cell multiplication and tumors.

Salt: Contributes to tumor growth through the retention of water in the cells, thickens blood and slows down the transmission of oxygen to the cells. Breads, spaghetti, desserts, and high gluten food are all high in salt content.

White mushrooms or any sort of mold: Thought by some to be carcinogenic.

Alcohol: Can increase the risk of cancer of the mouth, throat, esophagus, stomach, and liver.

Cancer Fighting Foods

Pursue a high fiber diet that includes raw fruits and vegetables, oats, wheat and rice bran, brown and wild rice, asparagus, spinach, carrots, cabbage, cucumbers, celery, endive, grapes, nuts and seeds.

Suggested foods for Breakfast: Hot cereals: cream of wheat, old fashioned flakes, steel cut oats, cream of rice, millet, or rye flakes. Use unbleached cane sugar, maple syrup, or unsulphured molasses to sweeten. Add ground cinnamon, unsulphured raisins. Freshly squeezed fruit juice, goat's milk, plain yogurt (with live Acidophilus), herb tea.

French toast (organic sprouted bread) with pure maple syrup, fruit, plain yogurt pancakes with pure maple syrup, bananas.

Lunch and dinner: Organic salad greens, steamed yellow and green vegetables, fish (many fish come from contaminated waters these days, so see if you can find a reliable source). Beef, chicken or turkey should be thoroughly cooked, organically raised and free range. Soup (preferably home made or use a brand that is not in an aluminum can), potatoes, boiled or baked.

Fresh vegetable or fruit juice: Carrot, beet, cabbage, apple, celery, spinach, grape, papaya, comfrey.

Seeds and Nuts (high in laetrile): Wheat grass, apricot, prune and peach pits, almonds, apple seeds, buckwheat.

Herbal teas

Chamomile: Reduces stress, aids sleep, digestion.

Cinnamon: Stimulates interferon production.

Comfrey: Healer.

Ginseng: Immunity.

Golden Seal: Tumor fighter and antibiotic.

Licorice: Interferon.

Pau D'arco: Tumor fighter.

POTENTIAL ENVIRONMENTAL HAZARDS

Chemicals: Please be aware that many products sold for home use such as cleaning products, paints and paint thinners, and bug sprays are potentially carcinogenic (cancer causing). Just having them in your living space letting off fumes can be as harmful as contact. Also eliminate asbestos from your home. Get natural cleaning products such as baking soda, borax, Bon Ami, white vinegar, and lemon juice. Use water based-paints and finishes. Get in the habit of reading labels.

Water: Chlorine, which is commonly used to treat water, can produce by-products that have proven to be potentially cancer causing. Water can also contain lead from old pipes and solder as well as harmful chemicals from industrial and agricultural pollution. Buy a reputable filter for the whole house if you can afford it or at least for your shower heads and kitchen faucet. Bathing can be as hazardous as drinking.

Light: Artificial light is everywhere: shopping malls, grocery stores, our homes, offices, and schools. Fluorescent bulbs lack the full spectrum we normally receive from sunlight. Photobiologist Dr. John Nash believes that full spectrum lighting is vitally important to our health for many reasons, including improved immunity. Limited spectrum lighting has also been associated with SAD (Seasonal Affect Disorder) syndrome which leads to depression. And many people would not be caught outdoors without products that block out the full spectrum, including sunglasses and sun block creams. These prevent us from receiving beneficial nutrients, such as vitamin D, from the sun. Full spectrum bulbs can be purchased to replace the regular bulbs in one's home. Proper lighting along with walks outside can be very beneficial to health and healing.

E.M.F.s: Electromagnetic fields are the radiation caused by high energy electrical or electronic activity. Avoid liv-

near high voltage power lines if you can. Don't sit ɔ close to TV's and microwave ovens, and if you use computer, obtain a shield for it. Office supply catalogs and retail stores carry various brands.

Personal Hygiene

Teeth: Many dentists who consider themselves 'holistic' no longer use silver amalgam fillings which contain mercury, a potentially toxic metal. If you can afford it, consider having your old silver fillings replaced.

Cosmetic and Body Care: Unfortunately, many products that call themselves 'natural' contain ingredients that are potentially harmful. Simple is best. The skin is the largest active organ in the body and can absorb great quantities of whatever is put on it. Again, educate yourself and read the labels.

IMAGERY

Using imagination in an active, yet relaxed and focused, state of mind can be a very effective technique for alleviating pain and dis-ease. Similar to both meditation and hypnosis, a person can use creative visualization to imagine oneself in a soothing, relaxing environment or activity. I like to envision myself lying in the shallow part of the ocean looking up at the deep blueness of the sky and feeling the waves lapping gently around my body. Choose a place or activity that invokes peace, safety and confidence. Imagine as many details as you can of how this would feel and look. Do not underestimate the power of this simple exercise.

Carl Simonton, M.D., and his wife Stephanie Matthews Simonton, trained cancer patients to supplement their regular therapy with imagery. They learned to visualize the cancer cells in their body being overwhelmed by their treatment and flushed out of their bodies. These people achieved a survival rate fully twice the national norm. Those who did die lived an average of a year and one half longer then the norm.

There is a similar technique in yoga where one visualizes healing white light streaming into the body while breathing in deeply. Negative energy is then visualized as expelled with each exhalation.

EXERCISE

Besides being generally healthy for everyone, moderate amounts of exercise may lower levels of circulating estrogen in women and thus help prevent cervical, breast and uterine cancer.

One of the simplest exercises, walking, is one of the best because it is gentle and yet profound in its benefit. For those who don't have time for an energetic walk each day, aerobic exercises such as running and aerobic dance may fit the bill. They are called aerobic because they elevate the breath and heart rates and cause the body to process much oxygen.

Rebounding (jumping) on a mini trampoline is a cellular exercise, helping to purge the lymphatic system of toxins. Many years of research has been confirmed by Dr. Kenneth Cooper's Institute of Aerobics Research, U.S. Air Force, NASA and Hong Kong University (see resources section under Albert E. Carter's book, *The New Miracles of Rebound Exercise*).

Regular exercise can also be a meditation with powerful stress-reducing potential. It's one of the best things a person can do for themselves.

Tibetan Five Rites

The five Tibetan rites help normalize hormone production along with many other benefits. They were introduced to the West by a retired British army colonel who discovered the much fabled and sought after "Fountain of Youth" at a remote monastery in the Himalayas. The rites enhance the flow of the subtle but powerful life force that circulates through the reproductive, adrenal, thymus, thyroid, pineal, and pituitary glands.

Each rite is done as many times as is comfortable at first and then the number of repetitions is gradually built up to twenty-one per day. While doing the exercises, it is extremely beneficial to breathe in deeply through the nose, and exhale with vigor through the mouth during each repetition.

THE FIRST RITE

Stand and spin clockwise at least 12 times. Your arms are extended straight out to the sides. This enhances the flow of life force through the body. Initially you may feel dizzy. One way to keep from getting dizzy is to hold your arms out from your body and focus attention on the thumbs.

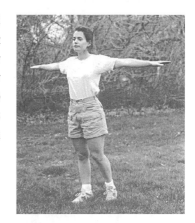

THE SECOND RITE

Lie on your back with your arms to your sides. The head lifts to the chest while the legs extend straight up into the air. Then lower the head and legs. At first this movement may seem difficult for you to keep the legs straight, however, with time you will improve and find it much easier. It is important to use the breath with all of these exercises. Concentrate on the abdominal region rather than from the chest.

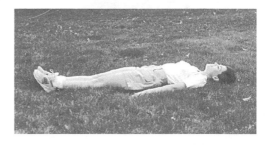

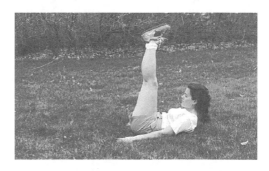

Breathe in deeply through the nose as you raise the legs and exhale through the mouth as you lower the legs.

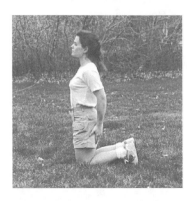

Kneel on the floor with your arms by your side with the hands placed against your thighs.

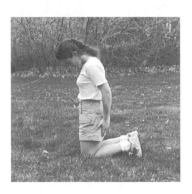

Bend the head forward while tucking the chin against your chest.

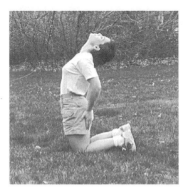

Then reverse the bend by bringing your head back toward your feet. Your hands on your thighs will help to support this movement. Then straighten out your head so it is aligned with your body. Breathe in with the backward arch., breathe out as your straighten.

Sit on the floor with your legs straight out and your feet twelve inches apart. Place the palms of your hands on either side of your buttocks. Tuck the chin in toward your chest.

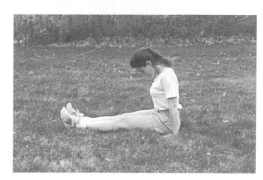

Then drop the head backwards at the same time raising your body and keeping the legs bent.

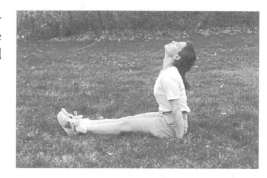

The trunk of the body should be in a straight line with the upper legs. First tense your muscles, then relax by coming back to the seated position. Breathe in as your body is lifted and out as your lower your body. The raised body

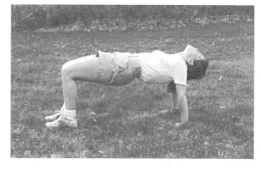

will resemble a table top with the arms and legs representing the four legs of the table.

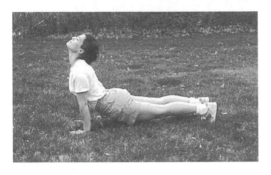

Begin with your body face down on the floor. Your arms and legs will support you. The arms and feet should be two feet apart and kept straight. Start perpendicular to the floor, then arch the spine and throw your head back as far as possible.

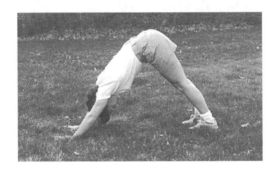

Then bend at the hips and bring your body back, tucking the chin into the chest. This position will resemble an inverted V. Breathe in deeply as you raise the body, breathe out as you lower it.

The rites can be done any time during the day. For best results, it is good to perform them six days a week. You can do a set in the morning, and then again later in the day to build up to the twenty-one. These rites are meant to enhance your entire system, so relax and enjoy. It is suggested not to take a cold bath immediately after the exercises.

Author's note: I have performed these rites for many years now and find them to be strengthening my whole body as well as the organs. I also have a tremendous amount of energy during the day.

Material from the Five Rites is reprinted from *Ancient Secret of the Fountain of Youth*, © 1989, with permission from Harbor Press, Box 1656, Gig Harbor, WA 98335. All rights reserved.

CHAPTER SEVEN

The Nuts and Bolts of Cancer and Essiac Therapy

by Dr. Jim Chan

"Medicine is not only a science,

but also the art of letting

our own individuality interact

with the individuality of the patient."

Albert Schweitzer

*I*n recent years I treated a number of cancer patients with Essiac. At first, I had to call the Emergency Drugs Release Program of Health and Welfare Canada to obtain authorization before getting the herbal compound from the Resperin Corporation. Then an article appeared in the *Vancouver Sun* covering several incredible stories of cancer remission with Essiac. The article was reprinted often and widely circulated. Since then, a number of products having similar composition came on the market place; some with a great deal of publicity and some through multi-level marketing techniques. As a result, Essiac has become a household word and one can probably walk down to the local health product outlet and purchase it freely.

IS ESSIAC EFFECTIVE?

Has Essiac been as effective as claimed in some of the sensational stories? Answering this question has been the goal of Resperin Corporation and Mankind Research Foundation for some time. Research efforts had been difficult due to lack of funding and support. The only source of funding, which is through sale of the compound, was greatly dampened by the corrosion of the market share by the flood of similar products. Based on the observation of thousands of cancer cases, I have not found Essiac to be effective across the board. However, there were cases that showed promising results. The majority of the cases needed other forms of support and intervention. Then why is it even worthwhile looking at Essiac as a possible therapy for cancer? First let us take a hard look at what we are dealing with in the disease called CANCER.

CANCER

The word cancer means crab. The ancient physicians observed masses in bodies that resembled the shape of crabs with tentacles reaching beyond the boundaries of organs and cavities. These were actually invasive arms of the tumor. Cancer is the uncontrolled multiplication and disorganized growth of cells forming a tumor that should not normally be in an organism. Cancer cells infiltrate and destroy adjacent tissues. Eventually, they gain access to the circulatory system and implant themselves in distant parts of the body. Cancer cells are typically growing at a faster rate than normal cells. The depletion of nutrients and high level of toxic waste in conjunction with the mechanical obstruction will ultimately destroy the host.

All of our cells have the ability to multiply if given the right signal to do so. The first cell that we came from, the zygote or fertilized egg, has an urgent need to multiply. Imagine developing a nine-pound tumor in nine months' time. This growth is commanded by a gene called the protooncogene. The initial stage of fetal development is very similar to the growth of a cancer. Fortunately, organized growth or differentiation kicks in at an appropriate time and we end up with parts of our body capable of specialized functions instead of looking like a big tumor.

Some scientists, including Dr. Govallo of Russia, have postulated that cancer could be treated like an abnormal fetal growth. The command for normal growth is stopped once we become a developed organism. This is achieved by the activation of the oncosuppressor gene which has the job of suppressing any gene expression of the protooncogene.

"Not all tumors are cancerous or malignant, some tumors have a close to normal growth rate and are considered to be benign."

In the case of cancer, the protooncogene becomes the oncogene, which effectively is the ultimate physical cause of cancer. The oncogene tends to stimulate cell growth in an unorganized fashion. Not all tumors are cancerous or malignant, some tumors have a close to normal growth rate and are considered to be benign.

The transformation of protooncogene to oncogene is referred to as oncogenesis, the birth of a cancer cell. It takes an average of eighty-five to two hundred days for cancer cells to progress one generation (some cancers can have a doubling time as fast as eight days and some as slow as seven hundred days). Clinical detection is limited to tumors the size of one centimeter or about ten billion cells. A tumor is already at its twenty-third generation at this clinically detectable size.

> "We can see how nature allows us a lot of time to do something about reversing the progression of the tumor load."

The human organism theoretically will not survive the existence of a tumor of the thirtieth generation in the body. We can see how nature allows us a lot of time to do something about reversing the progression of the tumor load. When cells transform, they almost always have markings that allow our immune system to detect and destroy them. Just like a fetus, however, if the tumor is allowed to grow to a certain size, the cancer cells will start to protect themselves by making themselves invisible to the immune system. They will even make their own growth stimulation factors.

Radiation and Cancer

There are various ways the oncogene can be activated. As we stand within the supposedly safe environment in our home, we are actually being bombarded by background radiation showering down from outer space. This radiation causes mutations of our DNA sequences. Repair of these mutations by our immune system takes place continuously. Sometimes, though, our bodies have a hard time keeping up.

Nowadays, our bodies must also contend with strong ionizing fields such as those generated by microwaves, electrical circuits and electronic devices. We are also frequently exposed to chemical mutagens such as pesticides and food additives, along with viral vectors, such as herpes, Epstein Barr, hepatitis, and human papilloma. All of these are capable of splicing a piece of genetic material into our DNA sequence or suppressing the oncosuppressor gene enough to activate the oncogene. When a cell is transformed, the surveillance team of the immune system—the natural killer cells—will quickly recognize the abnormal cell and destroy it. Theoretically, a tumor load of about one thousand cells is quite normal and our immune system can handle it without any extraordinary effort. At a tumor load of about 100,000 to 1 million cells, however, the body will start to feel the burden.

Stress and Cancer

Dr. Candice Pert of the National Institutes of Health found a link between stress and the functioning of the immune system. Stress actually weakens our immune function by causing the body to make a high level of neuropeptides that suppress the immune system. Most cancer patients can relate back to their social history and find the triggering factor that precedes the down turn of their health.

> "Most cancer patients can relate back to their social history and find the triggering factor that precedes the down turn of their health."

Ideally, cancer needs to be dealt with before clinical detection. Preventive strategies, such as stress management and avoiding carcinogenic agents, allow the body to keep up with the DNA repair mechanism and immune capability. From statistics coming from all sources, we know that cancer incidence is on the rise. We can go to the moon yet we seem helpless in our attempts to control one single gene expression.

Mainstream vs. Traditional Remedies

In the war against cancer, modern medicine has become skewed toward destructive procedures such as surgery, chemotherapy and radiotherapy. A number of surveys have shown the results of this approach to be disappointing. Many traditional remedies, however, have shown promise in controlling cancer. In Australia, for example, a common plant called Kangaroo apple was developed into a medicine that [may help] skin cancers. In India, urine therapy was practiced for thousands of years, and just recently, Dr. Bryzinski of Texas developed a promising medicine called Anti-neoplastin from human urine. Essiac is an herbal compound from the rich culture of the Native Americans that showed promising results right at our doorstep.

THE ESSIAC FORMULA

The Essiac formula was handed over to Resperin Corporation in 1977 by Rene Caisse on the recommendation of Mr. Chris Roman, a well respected businessman in Ontario. Rene Caisse insisted on the formula not be disclosed and it is still under lock and key today.

Burdock

The bulk of Essiac is burdock root, also called Artium lappa. Burdock is a plant that grows in many parts of the world. In Japan, burdock root is called "gobo" and is used in a delicious soup. In China, both the root and seed are used medicinally. In recent years, Japanese scientists found that burdock root contained a compound that reduced cell mutation. Fresh burdock root contains the polysaccharides arctose and inulin, which is capable of inducing differentiation in some cancer cells. One can easily estimate, therefore, that inulin is the major ingredient of the Essiac tea.

A number of polysaccharides in nature such as lentinin in shiitake mushrooms have been shown to have modulating effects on natural killer cell activities. Inulin is one of these glucans that could have similar effect. Though not directly proven, there were unpublished data from Resperin Corporation that showed Essiac having an enhancing effect on natural killer cell activities. Inulin also acts on insulin receptor sites. An herb called dahlia, containing very high level of inulin, is useful in diabetic patients to increase insulin receptor sensitivity. The presence of inulin reduces the requirement of insulin. Insulin is an endocrine hormone that also acts as a growth factor for cells. Perhaps by minimizing insulin response, the body is spared one of the many stimulating factors of tumor growth.

Turkey Rhubarb

The next ingredient in Essiac is turkey rhubarb, an herb that has demonstrated anti-tumor activity in animal tests. The ingredient that has anti-tumor activity is likely the glycoside that resembles Rhamnosyl-methoxylutcolin which is found in the Asian version of rhubarb. In Australia, Dr. Bill Chan discovered a glycoside in Kangaroo apples which has been incorporated in a medicine called "Curederm" that is very effective in treatment of skin cancers. Apparently, when a cancer cell picks up the sugar moiety of the glycoside, the alkaloid group is brought into the cytosol of the cancer cell. The alkaloid could initiate the lysis of hydrogen peroxide containing lysosomes in the cancer cell destroying the cancer cell internally.

Sheep Sorrel and Slippery Elm

The next ingredient, sheep sorrel, also contains alkaloids that may play a part in the cytotoxic activity. The fourth ingredient in Essiac, slippery elm, is primarily used in herbal medicine as a demulcent. It may serve primarily as a protective agent for the mucous lining against the alkaloids.

The Bottom Line

There are several different products on the market claiming to be either identical, similar or improved from the original Essiac formula. I have heard of anecdotal reports of positive results from all of these products. One particular product was claimed to have been improved by Rene Caisse after the formula was handed over to Resperin Corporation in 1978. We know that Rene Caisse left us in 1978 and hardly anything was done about Essiac. Whether we want to use Essiac treatment as an adjunctive or primary treatment, one may be wise to get the word from the horse's mouth. And with all the talk about how to deal with cancer, prevention through management of stress and a healthy life style is still the best cure and has the least human cost.

Dr. Jim C. Chan is a Naturopathic Physician practicing in Vancouver, British Columbia, Canada. Dr. Chan is a graduate of Bastyr University, where he serves on the board of directors. He currently sits on the subcommittee of Naturopathic Medicine of the Medical Service Commission of the Province of British Columbia. He is a past vice president of the Association of Naturopathic Physicians of British Columbia and a founding member of the American Association of Naturopathic Physicians and a member of Association of Acupuncturists of British Columbia.

Prior to establishing his Naturopathic practice, Dr. Chan received training in traditional Chinese Medicine in Hong Kong and China. His father, Dr. Chan Ching Lam, a Chinese herbalist who practiced for over fifty years, had great influence on him. Dr. Chan also trained and worked for a number of years in medical technology as well as research enzymology.

Dr. Chan taught Chinese Herbal Medicine at Bastyr University and helped found their Acupuncture program. He focuses on cancer treatments using biological medicine and oxidative therapies. Essiac has been a part of his practice for the past seven years.

CHAPTER EIGHT

The Possible
Missing Ingredient

by Christopher Gussa, Clinical Herbalist

"This formula is a gift from the Ojibwa to all mankind, all races, anyone! Why can't everyone just say thank you and accept it?"

Ojibwa Medicine Man

*A*lthough I had known about the "Essiac" formula for about 15 years I hadn't bothered to research it much until an older man came to me with some heart problems. While going through some diagnostics with him he explained that he had been[treated for effects] of prostate cancer by taking the Essiac formula and receiving a lot of prayer from family and friends. Up until that time I witnessed only about 1 out of 4 people being healed from this formula so I had to ask him, "where did you get your herbs and how much did you take?" He pulled out an old wrinkled up piece of paper from his wallet and said, "when I was out in California I went to see a naturopathic doctor, he gave me this list of herbs and told me if I or anyone else had any questions we could call him." The next day I gave this doctor a call.

It turned out this doctor was a very caring older man in his late 80's. We had a very nice conversation and he told me he was half Ojibwa Indian and that his father's father's were all Ojibwa Medicine Men from Ontario. He explained that he decided to practice in a white man's environment in L.A. but that he never lost the meaning of belonging to the Midewiwin. Anyway, he went on to say that he was saddened by all the commercial "hype" and bickering over who has the rights to this formula and had to laugh saying "I even call it the 'Essiac' formula most of the time."

But what I remember so fondly is when he said, "this formula is a gift from the Ojibwa to all mankind, all races, anyone! Why can't everyone just say thank you and accept it?"

I asked about the proportions of the four herbs and the dosages and he explained it to me as follows:

"I use a big handful of chopped, dried Burdock Root (my hands are kind of big, this weighs about 3 ounces). Then I use a big handful of chopped dried Sheep Sorrel herb (this weighs about 1 ounce). Then I use big pieces of dried Rhubarb Root amounting to about 1/2 ounce total (I use big pieces so the laxative effect is not boiled away). Then I add a wad of dried Slippery Elm (inner bark) about the size of a golf ball (this won't even move most scales, maybe 1/18 of an ounce). This makes a one week's supply, so boil it for about 15 minutes in one gallon of water then let it soak overnight in the gallon of water, strain it and store it in a one gallon apple juice jug in your fridge.

Drink one 8 ounce cup twice a day (or more if you feel like it). Don't dilute it, that's some kind of "wimpy, white man health food store" thinking. It tastes kind of thick and slippery—if you heat it do it on a burner in a small sauce pan. Don't ever heat it in a microwave or it will be useless. By the way, when you drink it pray that your body will get back in harmony with the Great Spirit."

After he told me all about the formula, he added that sometimes when tumors are very stubborn you have to use Blood Root along with the formula. I grinned to myself when I heard this because up until then I had been seeing my most success against cancer with a formula containing Blood Root (Chaparral, Red Clover, Dandelion Root, Yellow Dock Root, Burdock Root and Blood Root). The thought occurred to me to use the full strength traditional "Ojibwa Tea" with a few drops of a strong Blood Root tincture in each cup.

Blood Root is tricky to use in large doses due to it's over-reaction threshold so the following is exactly what I enclose to anyone that needs to take it along with the Ojibwa brew.

Directions for Blood Root Usage

IMPORTANT: If you are using Blood Root tincture with Dragon's "Ojibwa Tea" please follow these instructions carefully:

Dosage: On the average 5-10 drops (NOT DROPPERS) 2 times a day with your "tea". However, your tolerable threshold must be found. To accomplish this, start with 5 drops. Increase dosage by 1 drop per day until nausea occurs. If nausea occurs before you reach 10 drops, then back down 1 drop and hold that dosage.

DO NOT UNDER ANY CIRCUMSTANCES EXCEED 10 DROPS

If nausea occurs with the initial 5 drops, then start with 1 drop and work your way to your tolerable dosage as outlined above.

If all you can tolerate is 1-2 drops try increasing dosage by 1 drop after a week's use. If you still can only handle 1-2 drops then that is all you need, and it is doing

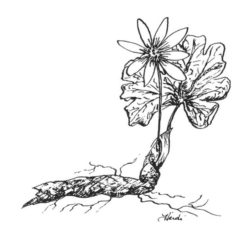

Bloodroot
Sanuinaria canadensis   Papaveracae (Poppy family)

Blood root is found in moist woods and near stream banks. Native to North America, from Quebec south to Florida and Texas and west to Kansas. This is a low growing perennial with a deep orange-red rhizome. Each flower bloom is enveloped in a single leaf. This leaf opens and enlarges as the single white flower blooms.

as well as 10 drops for someone else.

Blood Root is an extremely powerful substance. There are some (usually those who have a financial interest in chemotherapy, radiation or pharmaceutical companies) that say never take Blood Root internally, "it's way too dangerous" (and chemotherapy and radiation aren't?). However, we have observed no negative reactions in 100% of the hundreds of patients we have treated with Blood Root tincture when taken in these tolerable doses.

Since I have been using this combination at the Desert Dragon Healing Center, the results have been amazing. Here are a few case histories:

A woman (school teacher), 35 years old, had been diagnosed with non-Hodgkins Lymphoma. Her oncologist told her she had 2 years to live, there was nothing he could do. After coming to the Healing Center, she started the Ojibwa brew plus small amounts of Blood Root. After staying on the formula for just three weeks she felt much better. After two months she had a tumor marker test showing two-thirds lower markers. Six months later her tests showed absolutely normal and all her tumors are gone. She is staying on the formula in small doses for preventative reasons.

A woman, 60 years old, who had abdominal cancer had been treated with chemotherapy and radiation. After about two years it had come back in her liver and other organs. She came to the Healing Center mostly to inquire about the formula. She was to have a tumor marker test in three weeks. I convinced her to try the formula (with Blood Root). Her test showed one third lower markers and one month later two-thirds lower. Her oncologist said, "I don't know what you're doing but you certainly don't need chemo at this rate."

A man, about 40 years old, came to me with a large lump on his testicle and complained of passing blood. He did not see a doctor or get a biopsy (he explained his dislike for most doctors). I said "let's assume you have a cancerous situation (even if you don't) and get started on the formula." His lump went down in just a few days, he passed more blood after a week or so, then everything was normal. He stayed on the formula for about 3 months. It's been about 2 years and he's perfectly healthy.

A woman, 70 years old, had a large tumor in her mid colon area. She had it surgically removed. Her surgeon did not approve of chemotherapy or radiation and actually suggested she get on an herbal therapy. She had started on small amounts of "Essiac" but only half heartedly, frequently missing dosages. Several months later, they found large cancer spots on her liver. She came to the Desert Dragon Healing Center very frightened but finally willing to fight it aggressively. She started taking twice the dosage of what we normally suggest at the Center along with so much Blood Root that it frequently made her nauseous. She also immediately went from a diet of junk food to all organic vegetables, including lots of carrot juice. Her spots were completely gone in only two weeks, and her tumor markers are now lower than those of a typically healthy person.

A man, 35 years old, diagnosed with prostate cancer, came to the Center. He got started on the Ojibwa brew with Blood Root and found that 2 months later his tumor markers had not gone up but remained the same. He was taking some pharmaceutical drugs for arthritis pain and lots of Tylenol, etc. I advised him to quit taking all the pharmaceuticals if he could (because the brew just won't work the same with all that toxicity in his blood). He had recently moved to the coast and we were sending his herbs by mail. About three months later, I got a call from him saying his markers were almost normal. He told me he had found a good acupuncturist and he was able to get off his pain medication! (I've seen many similar cases where pharmaceuticals blocked the cure).

These are only a few of perhaps 50 cancer cases we have seen cured out of our little Healing Center alone. How many thousands of small clinics all over America have seen so much more? And when people like John F. Kennedy's personal doctor testify to the healing power of this formula, it becomes so obvious there must be a carefully organized cover up.

AFTERWORD

Essiac and the Hopi

A week before this book was headed out the door to the printers, I received a call from a friend who told me about Caroline, a woman in our community who has been brewing and delivering bottles of Essiac to give to some of the Hopis on Second Mesa in Arizona.

I called Caroline and told her about my Essiac book and asked if she would give me some details on how the Essiac was helping people on Second Mesa. She said she would be happy to talk with me and asked if I wanted to travel with her to Arizona. She was to bring Essiac to the Hopis in a few days. The timing was perfect since the following week the book was scheduled to be printed. Caroline said she would write letters to a couple of the Hopi men telling them about my book and asking if it would be all right for me to see and talk with them. She called me and said things were all set to go.

Caroline has always purchased the herbs and bottles from a local source. She brews the Essiac at home to take with her on her regular visits to the mesa. This time she was taking empty bottles and the herbs to show a Hopi man who had expressed interest in learning how to brew the Essiac for his village. Some of the Hopis were beginning to feel better and having good results from the herbs. More people were beginning to ask if they could have Essiac. It was time for Caroline to teach the Hopi man in the village how to brew the herbs to make the Essiac more readily available for others.

When we arrived at the Hopi mesa, we met the Hopi man who would be brewing the herbs. It seemed symbolic somehow that Caroline and I would be showing a Native American how to brew Essiac. The next day, which coincidentally happened to be a full moon, we prepared and started cooking the herbs in his family's kitchen. We didn't start preparing the Essiac mixture as early in the morning as we had planned to, so the bottles would have to be filled at midnight. That evening, with the moon lighting up the entire mesa, we stood in the kitchen pouring the warm Essiac liquid into the amber bottles. We had made enough Essiac to fill twelve 16-ounce bottles. We drank a small amount of the Essiac that was left, giving thanks for these special herbs. The experience is something Caroline and I will remember for a long time.

I was able to speak with two of the Hopi Elders; a woman and a man. They said that I could write of their experiences about Essiac. The talks weren't long, yet I was so grateful that they were willing to speak with me about the "medicine" they were taking.

Hopi Testimonies

Hopi Grandmother: She is in her late fifties and was recently diagnosed with diabetes. She is on the doctor's medicine. She started taking Essiac several months ago. One of her daughters prepares a tea with Essiac and distilled water in the morning and at bedtime. When the doctor tested her blood sugar recently, it had gone from over 300 to 130. Her energy is good. She enjoys taking the Essiac because it makes her feel better. Her legs get swollen at times, so she elevates them during the day and when she goes to bed. She feels the Essiac helps to keep the swelling down.

Hopi Elder: He has been on the Essiac for three months. Takes 1 tablespoon of the Essiac once a day. Before he started the Essiac, he had stomach problems. His stomach is much better and his energy is good.

Both of these people will continue on the Essiac. The Hopi who is preparing the herbs will continue to give the Essiac to people on the mesa.

I consider this experience with the Hopi as a blessing. I am grateful to have met them, and to know they are happy to take the "medicine."

Thank you Caroline for the heartfelt contribution you have given to the Hopi as well as to me.

Shortly after being diagnosed 1 1/2 years

ago with breast cancer, a friend shared

the Essiac book with me. It gave me the

hope that I could win this battle, and the

knowledge of how and where to begin.

Essiac is the key ingredient to my battleplan.

My husband and several friends are also taking

Essiac as a preventative measure.

I have also shared the Essiac book with many

others who have also benefited greatly.

Dollie Lucas

GLOSSARY OF TERMS

Alkaloid: an organic compound found in plants.

Anthelmintic: the property of destroying or expelling worms.

Artose: a complex sugar.

Cytotoxic: cell destroying.

Crysophanic Acid: an organic acid.

Decoction: A liquid preparation made by boiling a medicinal with water, usually one part plant to twenty parts water, boiled in a covered nonmetal container for about fifteen minutes.

Demulcent: a soothing agent.

Diaphoretic: A substance that increases perspiration.

Diuretic: An agent that increases the volume and flow of urine, thereby cleansing the excretory system.

Glucans: complex sugars that humans cannot digest.

Glycoside: an organic compound that has a sugar attached to it.

Infusion: The extraction of the active properties of a substance by steeping or soaking it, usually in water.

Inulin: a complex sugar that humans cannot digest.

Lentinin: a complex sugar.

Lysis: the destruction of a cell.

Lysosomes: bubbles in a cell that contain destructive compounds.

Neuropeptides: amino acid chains made by the brain.

Oncogene: a gene that causes cancer.

Oncogenesis: the formation of cancer cells.

Oncosuppressor: a gene that activates the cancer causing gene.

Oxalic Acid: an organic acid.

Papilloma: a lesion caused by a certain virus.

Periderm: the corky layer of the stem and tissues of the turkey rhubarb.

Petiole: the slender stalk by which the leaf is attached to the stem; leaf stalk.

Poltice: a substance applied on the surface of the body.

Polysaccharides: complex sugars.

Root stock: the root and its associated growth buds, used as a stock in plant preparation.

Refrigerant: a compound used to lower temperature.

Rhamnsyl Methoxy Lutcolin: a glycoside.

BIBLIOGRAPHY

The American Indians: People of the Lakes. Time-Life Books, 1994.

Bracebridge Examiner: "ESSIAC - A Cancer Remedy?" Bracebridge, Ontario, Canada. Series of 16 articles published beginning January, 1979, including: "Losing the Cancer War," by Dr. Samuel Epstein and Ralph Moss, and a testimonial letter by David Widdifield of Saabichton, BC, Canada, dated January 10, 1992.

Britton, Ted. "1981 Post-Gazette Humanitarian Award - Dr. Charles Armao Brusch." *Post-Gazette* newspaper, Boston, MA, Dec. 18, 1981.

Burton Goldberg Group. *Alternative Medicine.* Puyallup, WA: Future Medicine Publishing, Inc., 1993.

Buzenberg, Ann. "Can Native Herbs Cure Cancer?" *Spectrum Holistic News Magazine*, Vol. 32, September/October 1993, p. 21.

Caisse, Rene M., RN. *I Was Canada's Cancer Nurse.* Bracebridge, Ontario, Canada, 1980.

Carter, Albert E. *The Cancer Answer.* Fountain Hills, AZ: ALM Publishers, 1988.

Carter, Albert E. *The New Miracles of Rebound Exercise.* Fountain Hills, AZ: ALM Publishers, 1988.

Clark, Hulda Regehr, PhD, ND. *The Cure For All Cancers*. San Diego, CA: ProMotion Publishing, 1993.

Glum, Gary, DC. *Calling of An Angel*. Los Angeles, CA: Silent Walker Publishing, 1988.

Kelder, Peter. *Ancient Secret of the Fountain of Youth*. Harbor, WA: Harbor Press, Inc., 1985.

Kroeger, Hanna. *Parasites: The Enemy Within*. Boulder, CO: Hanna Kroeger Publications, 1991.

Livingston, Robert. *The Cancer Parasite*. Birmingham, AL.

Moss, Ralph. *The Cancer Industry*. New York, NY: Equinox Press, 1992.

Robinson, Elizabeth. "ESSIAC: An Interview with Dr. Gary Glum." Excerpted from *Wildfire*, Vol. 6, No. 1, February 1993. Reprinted with permission from *Omni Magazine*.

Santillo, Humbart, ND, MH. *Food Enzymes: The Missing Link to Radiant Health and Intuitive Eating*. Prescott, AZ: Hohm Pres, 1987.

Snow, Sheila (Fraser), and Allen, Carroll. "Could ESSIAC Halt Cancer?" *Homemaker's Magazine*, June-August, 1977.

Snow, Sheila. "ESSIAC: Exploring the Controversial Cancer Formula." excerpted from the *Canadian Journal of Herbalism*, Summer 1991.

Snow, Sheila. *The Essence of Essiac*. Port Carling, Ontario, Canada, 1993.

Stainsby, Mia. "Cancer Hope Reborn." *Sedona Journal of Emergence*, April 1993. Excerpted from the *Vancouver Sun*, May 16, 1992.

Thomas, Richard. "The Essiac Report." *Alternative Treatment Information Network*, Los Angeles, CA, 1993.

Valentine, Tom. "A Special Report: ESSIAC: An Herbal Treatment for Cancer." For Associated Partners West. Copyright 1989, S. J. Corinth Corp., Iowa City, IA. (Including an article about D. Emma Carson)

Vecsey, Christopher. *Traditional Ojibwa Religion and its Historical Changes.* The American Philosophical Society, Vol. 152. Philadelphia, PA., 1983.

Walters, Richard. *Options: The Alternative Cancer Therapy Book.* Garden City Park, NY: Avery, 1994.

Weil, Andrew, MD. *Natural Health, Natural Medicine.* Boston, MA: Houghton Mifflin Co., 1990.

Werbach, Melvyn R., MD. *Nutritional Influences on Illness.* New Canaan, CT: Keats Publishing, Inc., 1990.

RESOURCES

Bracebridge Public Library
94 Manitoba Street
Bracebridge, P1L 2B5
Ontario, Canada
Nancy Summerly, Research Librarian

Center for Advancement in Cancer Education
Susan Silberstein, Ph.D., Executive Director
300 E. Lancaster Avenue, Ste 100
Wynnewood, PA 19096 tel.: (610) 642-4810
Newsletter, scientific articles, books, tapes.
e-mail: onconurs@bellatlantic.net
www.beatcancer.org

Eden Acres
Organic Network
12100 Lima Center Road
Clinton, MI 49236-9618 tel.: (517) 456-4288
International Directory of Organic Resources $15
Directory (by state) of farmers, alternative medicine, resources, natural clothing
and suppliers of organic food.
e-mail: jean@lni.net

Exceptional Cancer Patients
522 Jackson Park Drive
Meadville, PA 16335 tel.: (814) 337-8192 fax: (814) 337-0699
Books, tapes, and listing of imagery professionals.
www.ecap-online.org

Health Quarters Ministries
955 Garden of the Gods Rd.; Ste C
Colorado Springs, CO 80907 tel.: (719) 593-8694
Non-profit resource center. Offers eleven-day lodging for renewal of health and
spirit.

Herb Research Foundation
1007 Pearl Street, Ste. 200
Boulder, CO 80302 tel.: (303) 449-2265 fax: (303) 449-7849
Research information.
www.herbs.org

Kripala Yoga
Himalayan Institute of Yoga Science and Philosophy
Rt. 1, Box 400
Honesdale, PA 18431 tel.: 1-800 822-4547
Catalogue of books, videocassettes, and yoga centers.

Mind/Body Health Sciences, Inc.
393 Dixon Road
Boulder, CO 80302-3138 tel.: (303) 440-8460
Annual news letter.

Carolyn Myss, Ph.D.
Sounds True Catalog
413 Arthur Avenue
Louisville, CO 80027 tel.: 1-800 333-9185
Energy anatomy.
www.soundstrue.com

Nature's Best Distributors
16508 E. Laser Drive, Bldg. B
Fountain Hills, AZ 85268 tel.: 1-800 624-7114
Carries Albert Carter books, rebounders, vitamins.
www.naturesdistributers.com

Michael Rice, ND
Rt. 3, Box 3280
Theodosia, MO 65761 tel.: (417) 273-4891 fax: (417) 273-4522
Tapes, lectures on natural health and mind/body therapy.

The Health Resource, Inc.
Janice R. Guthrie, Director
933 Faulkner Street
Conway, AR 72032 tel.: (501) 329-5272; 1-800 949-0090
fax: (501) 329-9489
Information center.
www.thehealthresourse.com

Uchee Pines
30 Uchee Pines Road, Ste. 75
Seale, AL 36875-5702 tel.: (334) 855-4764 fax: (334) 855-9014
Hypothermia treatment, healing center for alternative treatments.

Vegetarian Times
#4 High Ridge Park
Stamford, CT 06905 tel.: (203) 321-1777 fax: (203) 322-1966
Magazine, general information, diet and menus for vegetarian lifestyle.
www.vegtimes.com

World Research Foundation
41 Bell Rock Plaza
Sedona, AZ 86351 tel.: (520) 284-3300
Large alternative medicine research library.
www.wrf.org

HERBAL ASSOCIATIONS

Organizations publishing newsletters and providing education about herbs.

American Botanical Council
P.O. Box 144345
Austin, TX 78714-4345 tel.: (512) 926-4900 fax: (512) 926-2345
www.herbalgram.org

American Herb Association
P.O. Box 1673
Nevada City, CA 95959-1673 tel.: (530) 265-9552 fax: (530) 274-3140
Quarterly newsletter.

American Herbal Products Association
8484 Georgia Ave. #370
Silver Springs, MA 20910 tel.: (301) 588-1171 fax: (301) 588-1174
www.ahpa.org

American Herbalists Guild
P.O. Box 70
Roosevelt, UT 84066 tel.: (435) 722-8434 fax: (435) 722-8452
www.healthy.net/herbalists

SUPPLIERS OF ESSIAC

Aphrodesia Products, Inc.
264 Bleeker Street
New York, NY 10014 tel.: (212) 989-6440
Tinctures, powders, capsules, herbs.

For Your Health Pharmacy
13758 Lake City Way, NE
Seattle, WA 98125-3616 tel.: 1-800 456-4325 fax: (206) 363-8790

Frontier Herbs
3021 78th Street / P.O. Box 299
Norway, IA 52318 tel.: 1-800 669-3275

Harvest Health Foods
1944 Eastern Avenue, SE
Grand Rapids, MI 49507 tel.: (616) 245-6268 fax: (616) 245-8034

Herb Products Company
P.O. Box 0898
North Hollywood, CA 91603 tel.: (818) 761-0351 fax: (818) 508-6567
Non-chemically treated herbs, some organic.

Herbs, Etc.
1340 Rufina Cr.
Santa Fe, NM 87505 tel.: (505) 471-6488 fax: (505) 471-0941

Indiana Botanical Gardens
3401 W. 37th Avenue
Hobart, IN 46342 tel.: 1-800 644-8327 fax: (219) 947-4148
www.botanichealth.com

InterNatural
P.O. Box 489
Twin Lakes, WI 53181
800-643-4221
email: internatural@internatural.com
website: www.internatural.com
Retail herbs, Essiac and other health products.

Kali Press
2222 Creekview St.
Carrollton, TX 75006
order line: 888-999-5254
email: mail@kalipress.com
website: www.kalipress.com
Wholesale and distributor inquiries welcome.
Essiac and other health products.

Lotus Light
P.O. Box 1008
Silver Lake, WI 53170
800-548-3824
email: lotuslight@lotuspress.com
website: www.lotuslight.com
Wholesale herbs, Essiac and other health products.

Marco Industries
3431 W. Thunderbird, Ste. 144
Phoenix, AZ 85023 tel.: 1-800 726-1612
Tinctures.

Spirit Mountain Botanicals
Attn: Kendra Whittaker, Clinical Herbalist
120 Sandia Circle, C.R. 520
Bayfield, CO 81122 tel.: (970) 884-9637
Herbs, Essiac formula.

Ojibwa Tea of Life
Michelle Kalevik (Reiki master, second degree)
P.O. Box 200041
Denver, CO 80220 tel.: (303) 322-7930 fax: (303) 316-3971
Tincture and books.

Winter Sun Trading Company
107 N. San Francisco, Ste. One
Flagstaff, AZ 86001 tel.: (520) 774-2884
Phyllis Hogan, Clinical Herbalist, Ethnobotanist
Herbs, tinctures.
www.wintersun.com

CLINICS

Alternative clinics are listed here as opportunities for individuals to educate themselves on the treatments each of these clinics provide. Healing involves a variety of different modalities, and the responsibility for illness and treatment remains with each person.

Bio-Medical Center
P.O. Box 433654
San Ysidro, CA 92143 tel.: 011 52 66-84-9011 (9081, 9082, 9376)
Hoxsey Therapy.

Burzynski Clinic
12000 Richmond Ave.
Houston, TX 77082 tel.: (281) 597-0111 fax: (281) 597-1166
www.cancermed.com/bri.htm

Cancer Control Society
2043 N. Berendo St. Los Angeles, CA 90027 tel.: (213) 663-7801
Alternative cancer treatment centers.

Dr. Jim Chan, N.D.
3380 Maquinna Drive, Suite 101
Vancouver, BC, Canada
V5S 4C6 tel.: (604) 435-3786 fax: (604) 436-2426

Desert Dragon Healing Center
P.O. Box 1735
Benson, AZ 85602 tel.: (520) 586-7955

The Gerson Institute
P.O. Box 430
Bonita, CA 91908-0430 tel.: (619) 472-7450
www.gerson.org

Nicholas Gonzales, M.D.
36A E 36th Street, Ste. 204
New York, NY 10016 tel.: (212) 213-3337 fax: (212) 213-3414
Kelly's Therapy.

International Medical Center
H. Ray Evers, M.D., Founder ('grandfather' of chelation therapy)
424 Executive Center Blvd., Ste 100
El Paso, TX 79902 tel.: (915) 584-0931 fax: (915) 534-0272
Diagnostic and therapeutic programs.

ALTERNATIVE MEDICAL ASSOCIATIONS

American Association of Naturopathic Physicians
601 Valley Street, Ste. 105
Seattle, WA 98109 tel.: (206) 298-0126 fax: (206) 298-0129

American Holistic Medical Association
6728 Old Village Drive
McLean, VA 22101 tel.: (703) 556-9728 fax: (703) 556-8729
www.holisticmedicine.org

Herbal Healer Academy
HC 32 Box 97-B
Mountain View, AR 72560 tel.: (870) 269-4177
Dr. Marijah McCain
Herbal products, training, catalog.
www.drherbs.com

Mankind Research Foundation, Inc.
1315 Apple Avenue
Silver Spring, MD 20910 tel.: (301) 587-8686 fax: (301) 587-8688
Producer and researcher of original Rene Caisse formula; carry capsule, liquid and
herbal tea kits, non-profit.
e-mail: uv@uvbi.com
www.uvbi.com

INDEX

IN GRATITUDE

*A portion of the proceeds
from the sale of this book
will be donated to
Native American study programs.*

More Titles from Lotus Press

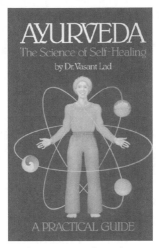

AYURVEDA: THE SCIENCE OF SELF-HEALING
Dr. Vasant Lad

175 pp pb $10.95   ISBN 978-0-9149-5500-9

For the first time a book is available which clearly explains the principles and practical applications of Ayurveda, the oldest healing system in the world. This beautifully illustrated text thoroughly explains history & philosophy, basic principles, diagnostic techniques, treatment, diet, medicinal usage of kitchen herbs & spices, first aid, food aid, food antidotes and much more.

More than 50 concise charts, diagrams and tables are included, as well as a glossary and index in order to further clarify the text.

Dr. Vasant Lad, a native of India, has been a practitioner and professor of Ayurvedic Medicine for more than 15 years. For the past four years he has conducted the only full-time program of study on Ayurveda in the United States as Director of The Ayurvedic Institute in Albuquerque, New Mexico. Dr. Lad has lectured extensively throughout the U.S. and has written numerous published articles on Ayurveda.

YOGA FOR YOUR TYPE
**Dr. David Frawley &
Sandra Summerfield Kozak, M.S.**

296 pp os • $29.95 • ISBN 978-0-9102-6130-2

This is the first book that details how to choose Yoga asanas (Yoga poses) most appropriate for your unique body type according to the five thousand year old system of Ayurvedic medicine. These two systems of healing and energy management have long been regarded as effective methods of relieving stress, creating personal balance, eliminating ailments, and relieving chronic pain. *Yoga for Your Type* presents a fundamental understanding of both Yoga and Ayurveda and provides the information needed for you to balance your energy and feel healthy.

"By reading this book, you will be able to personalize your yoga program and gain maximum benefit in integrating body, mind and spirit as one experience of consciousness."
— **Deepak Chopra, M.D.,** Author of *Grow Younger Live Longer*

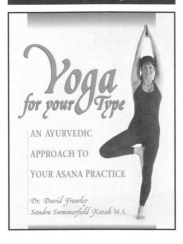

"Editors' Choice" – Yoga Journal

AN AYURVEDIC
APPROACH TO
YOUR ASANA PRACTICE

Dr. David Frawley
Sandra Summerfield Kozak M.S.

Other Titles from Lotus Press

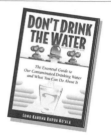

Don't Drink the Water:
The Essentail Guide to Our Contaminated Drinking Water and What You Can Do About It
Lono Kahuna Kupua Ho'ala

Additional copies of **Don't Drink the Water** are available through Lotus Press.

Trade Paper ISBN 978-0-9628-8829-8 112 pp $11.95

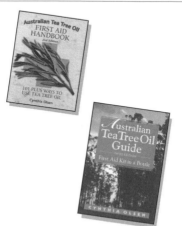

The Authoritative Tea Tree Oil Reference Books
Cynthia Olsen

Author/researcher Cynthia Olsen presents the most comprehensive books on this ancient remedy. The **Australian Tea Tree Oil First Aid Handbook** describes 101 ways to use tea tree oil (*Melaleuca alternifolia*) from head to toe—a must for users of this "first aid kit in a bottle." The new **Australian Tea Tree Oil Guide** contains updated information which includes production, quality control, research and a practitioners section.

Australian Tea Tree Oil First Aid Handbook, 2nd Edition
Trade Paper ISBN 978-1-8909-4102-4 96 pp $6.95

Australian Tea Tree Oil Guide, 3rd Edition
Trade Paper ISBN 978-1-8909-4101-7 140 pp $9.95

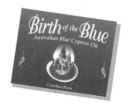

Birth of the Blue: Australian Blue Cypress Oil
Cynthia Olsen

A new, magnificent, aqua colored essential oil from the Northern Territory of Australia. Selected as the "Essence of the Sydney 2000 Summer Olympics." Blue Cypress Oil's woody fragrance has soothing and moisturizing skin benefits.

Trade Paper ISBN 978-1-8909-4104-8 88 pp $7.95

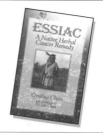

Essiac: A Native Herbal Cancer Remedy, 2nd Edition
Cynthia Olsen

The remarkable story of Canadian nurse Rene Caisse and her herbal anti-cancer formula.

Winner of the Small Press Book Award

Trade Paper ISBN 978-1-8909-4100-0 144 pp $12.50

Available at bookstores and natural food stores nationwide or order your copy directly by sending the cost of the book(s) plus $2.50 shipping/handling ($.75 s/h for each additional copy ordered at the same time) to:

Lotus Press, PO Box 325, Dept. STTG, Twin Lakes, WI 53181 USA

toll free order line: 800 824 6396   office phone: 262 889 8561   office fax: 262 889 2461
email: lotuspress@lotuspress.com   web site: www.lotuspress.com

Lotus Press is the publisher of a wide range of books and software in the field of alternative health, including Ayurveda, Chinese medicine, herbology, aromatherapy, Reiki and energetic healing modalities. Request our free book catalog.